Intermittent Fasting for Women Over 50

The Power of Fasting to Reset your Metabolism, Lose Weight
and Rejuvenate Yourself
Incl. Recipes and 28-Day Weight Loss Challenge

By Angela Burrows

Disclaimer

The recipes and information in this book are provided for educational and entertainment purposes only. Please always consult a licensed professional before making changes to your lifestyle or diet. The Author and publisher shall have neither liability nor responsibility to anyone with respect to any loss or damage caused or alleged to be caused directly or indirectly by the information contained in this book. All trademarks and brands within this book are for clarifying purposes only and are owned by the owners themselves, not affiliated with this document.

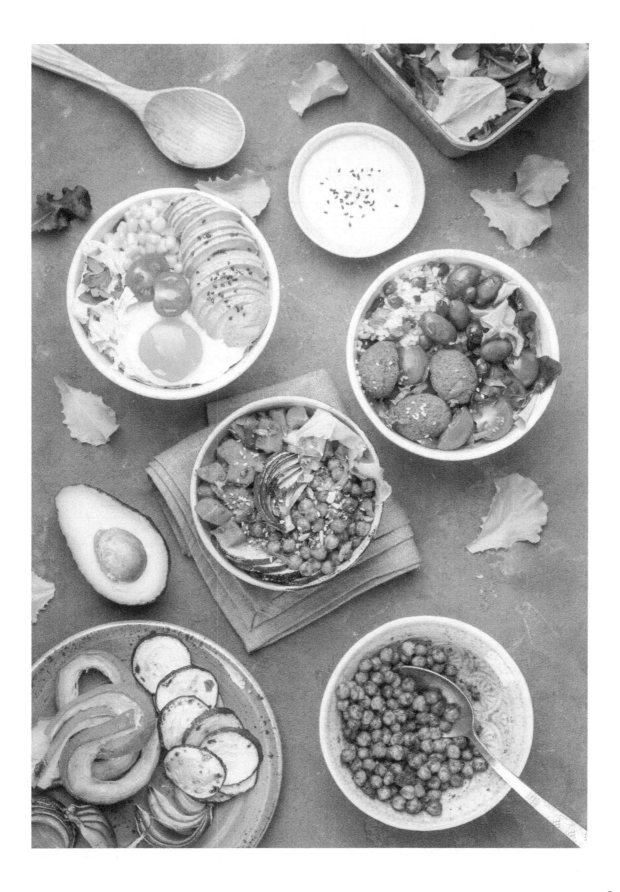

Table of Contents

INTRODUCTION

Intermittent fasting is an increasingly popular dietary strategy that has been around for centuries. I'll start this book with a general introduction to the concept, break down intermittent fasting as it pertains to different populations, and then give a couple of personal anecdotes.

What is intermittent fasting? Intermittent fasting can be defined as the practice of scheduling you are eating into narrow windows during the day. The windows maybe 4 or 6 hours long, or they could be 12 hours long. The eating window could be at night or first thing in the morning. The time is optional-- as long as you do it.

Who should do intermittent fasting? As with any dietary strategy, there are circumstances when it might not be the best choice for everyone. However, in my opinion, IF is a highly effective way to lose weight. It can also support healthy body composition (more muscle) and improve hormonal profile (less insulin). There are benefits for virtually all demographics (obese/overweight/etc.), although males may gain a bit fatter than females. It comes down to personal preference with regards to food timing and type. The purpose of this book is to outline the scientific underpinnings of intermittent fasting and provide some anecdotal case studies. Without getting too much into the weeds with nutrition science, I'll try to present the fundamental concepts as best I can. It won't be all-inclusive (as many other factors come into play regarding nutrition). All judgments regarding your situation should be made with professional assistance from a qualified medical or nutritional professional.

Intermittent Fasting for Women Over 50

Many women who are obese, over-weight, or pre-menopausal find it difficult to lose body fat. Long-term periods of calorie restriction (i.e., caloric deficit) in such cases leave many women feeling worse than they already did. Calorie restriction could also affect the pituitary gland, which secretes prolactin, a hormone that stimulates milk production and lactation in breastfeeding mothers. Prolactin is also the hormone that signals the uterus to stop producing lining cells (necessary for a pregnancy). For this reason, women tend to be more sensitive to calorie restriction than men are. As such, intermittent fasting can lead to a more significant loss of fat mass during periods of weight loss with a minor disadvantage than traditional calorie reductions.

Some women do pretty well on an intermittent fasting schedule, while others struggle. If you're male (over 55), you can still see benefits, although female physiology will probably favor IF even more so than men. Generally speaking, IF does not cause an increase in muscle loss, which is good news for most people (and especially women).

Studies show that if the calorie intake is too low, muscle loss will occur regardless of whether the fasted state was adhered to. I've been experimenting with IF for a few months now, and I can attest to its effectiveness for burning fat and increasing muscle mass.

What are the best fasts? Generally speaking, one of two categories is recommended: 16-hour fasts or 6-hour fasts – both in the morning. I've had success with the longer fast, but it was only successful during short periods. I don't think that a 24 hour fast or even a longer 12 hours fast would be necessary for most people.

It will walk you through all of the essential information you'll need to start intermittent fasting.

Chapter 1. BASICS OF INTERMITTENT FASTING

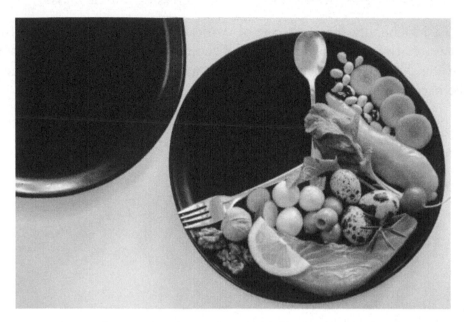

Intermittent fasting has been practiced for millennia for a variety of reasons. Although utilizing it mainly for weight reduction is a relatively recent practice. It has a long tradition of spiritual contact, disease prevention, enhancing focus, and reducing aging symptoms, among other items. Since the advent of agriculture, fasting has been practice by almost every faith, culture, and society.

Around 400 BC, Hippocrates, the founding father of modern medicine, used to recommend fasting. Nowadays, most people are aware of this strategy because of its proven potential to help people lose weight. Many popular diet plans emphasize when to eat instead intermittent fasting emphasizes what to eat.

Intermittent fasting fixes when eating during the day. Fasting for several hours per day or consuming just one meal a couple of times a week will aid in weight loss.

You don't have to give up your favorite snacks or consume fewer calories per meal to adopt the intermittent fasting lifestyle. Indeed, the most common form of intermittent fasting allows participants to miss breakfast before consuming two meals later in the day. This form of lifestyle modification is perfect for people having trouble keeping to a stricter eating schedule. It just takes a slight change to achieve significant differences, rather than being expected to change all at once. It renders intermittent fasting a perfect long-term and short-term option. It is simple to get started with and continue within the long run and reliable enough to provide consistent results, motivating those who follow it to keep up their successful work.

How Does Intermittent Fasting Work?

The effectiveness of intermittent fasting can be attributed to the undeniable fact that your body responds when eating than fasting separately.

This condition appears approximately five minutes after you finish your meal. It can last up to five hours, depending on the type of meal and how difficult it is for the body to convert it into energy. When the body is in this state, it actively produces insulin, making it far more challenging to burn fat than when produced insulin. Before fasting, the following condition occurs immediately after digestion.

It's called the buffer period. It will last from eight to twelve hours, depending on what you last ate and on your specific body chemistry. Your body will only burn fat at maximum productivity when in this environment until your insulin levels have returned to normal. Because of the duration of time needed to enter an actual fasting state, many people never witness the maximum impact because they barely go longer than eight hours without food, much less twelve. It isn't to say that such transition is impossible; what you must do is take advantage of this normal condition to break the three squares a day habit.

Intermittent Fasting Benefits

Intermittent fasting does more than burn fat, according to a study. "Changes with this metabolic switch affect the body and the brain," Mattson says. During intermittent fasting, several mechanisms happen to protect organs from chronic diseases: heart diseases, type 2 diabetes, age-related neurodegenerative conditions, inflammatory bowel disease, and many cancers. Knowing the advantages of intermittent fasting will inspire you to give it a shot.

Here are some of the effects of intermittent fasting that have been discovered so far through studies:

- Improved Cardiac Health: Lowering blood pressure and lowering LDL cholesterol increases heart health.
- Diabetes Management: Fasting reduces the incidence of diabetes. During fasting, decreased insulin levels, and the blood does not regulate blood glucose levels.
- Weight Loss: Since insulin levels are lower, accumulated fat may be used as energy, resulting in weight loss.
- Muscle mass increases as HGH (Human Growth Hormone) levels rise. The lean muscle mass increases as you pair fasting with exercise. Calorie burning is aid by increased muscle mass.
- Decreased Inflammation: Not eating decreases inflammation in the body dramatically. Since there is less insulin in the blood, the kidneys can remove extra salt and water from the body, decreasing inflammation.
- Lower Blood Pressure: Blood pressure is lower as the kidneys expel extra fluids and salt.

- Improved Well-Being: Fasting has psychological advantages such as a sense of balance, improved body image, and reduced stress.
- Faster Metabolism: As adrenalin levels rise, the metabolism accelerates.
- Eating Less: Fasting will help you shed weight spontaneously by stopping you from eating outside the fasting window.
- Delay in Aging and Disease: Fasting causes the body's cells to regenerate and work faster.
- Increased Cognitive Function: As you adopt a fasting regimen, your mental sharpness, and concentration increase.

Is Intermittent Fasting Safe?

Some people use intermittent fasting to lose some weight. Others use it to treat serious illnesses, including irritable bowel syndrome, elevated cholesterol, or arthritis. Intermittent fasting, on the other hand, isn't for all.

Before following intermittent fasting (or other diets), consult with your primary care physician. Some individuals should avoid experimenting with intermittent fasting:

- Children and teenagers under the age of eighteen.
- Women who are expecting a child or who are breastfeeding.
- People with diabetes and those with blood sugar concerns.
- People who have had an eating disorder in the past.

People who aren't in these groups can successfully do intermittent fasting, can continue the regimen forever as it's a lifestyle change with advantages.

Keep in mind that intermittent fasting may have a variety of consequences depending on the person. If you have unusual distress, headaches, nausea, or other signs after beginning intermittent fasting, consult your doctor.

Is Intermittent Fasting Good for Women?

Women are motivated to intermittent fasting for several factors, including:

- Improve lean muscle buildup
- A boost in energy
- Continuous weight loss
- An increased cellular stress response
- Oxidative stress and inflammation reduced
- Improve insulin sensitivity in overweight women
- Increased nerve growth factor development improves cognitive performance

Chapter 2. MENOPAUSE AND HORMONAL BALANCE

Menopause is one of the most challenging phases in a woman's life. When our bodies begin to change, and critical natural transitions occur, they are too often negatively affected. At the same time, it is essential to learn how to change our eating habits and eating patterns appropriately. It often happens that a woman is not ready for this new condition and experiences it with a feeling of defeat as an inevitable sign of time travel. This feeling of prostration turns out to be too invasive and involves many aspects of one's stomach.

Therefore, it is vital to remain calm as soon as there are messages about the first signs of change in our human body. Ward off the onset of menopause for the proper purpose and minimize the adverse effects of suffering, especially in the early days. Even during this challenging transition, targeted nutrition can be very beneficial.

What Happens to The Body of a Menopausal Woman?

A balanced diet - without significant weight fluctuations - will undoubtedly support women going through menopause We can distinguish between the pre-menopausal phase (around 45 to 50 years) physiologically compatible with a drastic reduction in the production of the hormone estrogen (responsible for the menstrual cycle, which starts irregularly This period corresponds to a series of complex and highly subjective endocrine changes such as headache, depression, anxiety, and sleep disorders.

When someone enters actual menopause, estrogen hormone production decreases even more dramatically. The range of the symptoms widens, leading to large amounts of the hormone, for example, to a particular class called catecholamine adrenaline. The result of these changes is a dangerous heat wave, increased sweating, and the presence of tachycardia, which can be more or less severe.

However, the changes also affect the female genital organs, with the volume of the breasts, uterus, and ovaries decreasing. The mucous membranes become less active, and vaginal dryness increases. There may also be changes in bone balance, with decreased calcium intake and increased mobilization at the expense of the skeletal system. Because of this, there is a lack of continuous bone formation, and conversely, erosion begins, which is a tendency for osteoporosis.

Although menopause causes relevant changes that significantly change a woman's body and soul, metabolism is the worst changement. In fact, during menopause, the absorption and accumulation of sugars and triglycerides change. It is easy to increase some clinical values such as cholesterol and triglycerides, which lead to high blood pressure arteriosclerosis. In addition, many women often complain of disturbing circulatory disorders and local edema, especially in the stomach. It also makes weight gain more frequent, even though you haven't changed your eating habits.

The Ideal Diet for Menopause

In cases where disorders related to the arrival of menopause become challenging to manage, drug or natural therapy under medical supervision may be necessary. The contribution given by a correct diet at this time can be considerable. In fact, given the profound variables that come into play, it is necessary to modify our food routine, both in order not to be surprised by all these changes and to adapt in the most natural way possible.

The drop in estrogen always causes the problem of fat accumulation in the abdominal area. It is also responsible for most women's classic hourglass shape, which consists of depositing fat mainly on the hips, which begins to fail with menopause. As a result, we go from a gynoid condition to an android one, with a fatty increase localized on the belly. In addition, it is reducing the metabolic rate of disposal. It means that even if you do not change your diet and eat the exact quantities of food as you always have, you could experience weight gain, which will be more marked in the presence of bad habits or an irregular diet. The digestion is also slower and intestinal function becomes more complicated. It further contributes to swelling and intolerance, and digestive disorders that have never been disturbed before. Therefore, the beginning will be more problematic and challenging to manage during this period. The distribution of nutrients must be different: reducing the amount of low carbohydrate, which is always preferred not to be purified, helps avoid the peak of insulin and at the same time maintains stable blood sugar.

Furthermore, it will be necessary to increase the quantity of both animal and vegetable proteins slightly; choose good fats, prefer seeds and extra virgin olive oil, and severely limit saturated fatty acids. All this to increase the proportion of antioxidants taken will help counteract the effect of free radicals, whose concentration begins to grow during this period. It will be necessary to prefer foods rich in phytoestrogens. It will help control the states of stress to which subjected, which will favor, at least in part, the overall estrogenic balance.

These molecules are classified into three main groups. The foods that contain them should never be missing on our tables: isoflavones, present mainly in legumes such as soy and red clover; lignans, of which flax seeds and oily seeds in general, are vibrant; coumestans, found in sunflower seeds, beans, and sprouts. A calcium supplementation will be necessary through cheeses such as parmesan, dairy products such as yogurt, egg yolk, and some vegetables such as rocket, Brussels sprouts, broccoli, spinach, asparagus; legumes; dried fruit such as nuts, almonds, or dried grapes.

Excellent additional habits that will help to regain well-being may be: limiting sweets to sporadic occasions, thus drastically reducing sugars (for example, by giving up sugar in coffee and getting used to drinking it bitterly); learn how to dose alcohol a lot (avoiding spirits, liqueurs, and aperitif drinks) and choose only one glass of good wine when you are in company, this because it tends to increase visceral fat which is what is going to settle at the level abdominal. Even by eating lots of fruit, it isn't easy to reach a high carbohydrate quota as in a traditional diet. However, a dietary plan to follow can be helpful to have a more precise indication of how to distribute the foods. One's diet must be structured personally, based on specific metabolic needs and one's lifestyle.

Chapter 3. INTERMITTENT FASTING TYPES

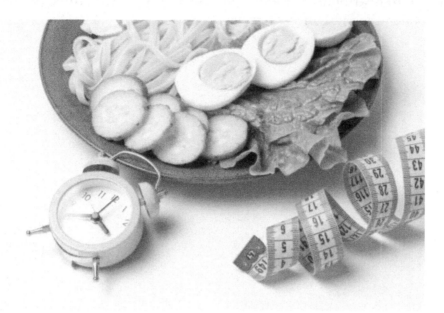

There are a variety of ways can do intermittent fasting. The number of fast days and calorie allowances differ between the approaches. Intermittent fasting entails going without food for a period, either entirely or partly, until eating normally.

According to research, this type of eating will help you lose weight, improve your fitness, and live longer. Intermittent fasting advocates claim that it is simpler to adhere to than conventional calorie-controlled diets. Intermittent fasting is a personal experience for each person, and different styles will match different people. Continue reading to learn about various types of intermittent fasting.

Lean-Gains Method

The lean-gain method has some alternative titles on the web, but its popularity stems from the idea that it helps people lose weight while still building muscle. Through diligent fasting, eating well, and exercising, you would shift all the fat into strength using the lean-gains method.

This strategy allows you to fast for 14 to 16 hours and then feed and work out for the remaining 10 or 8 hours of the day. Unlike crescendo, this approach requires regular fasting and feeding rather than alternated days of fasting and eating. Start with a 14-hour fast and work your way up to 16 if you're relaxed with it, but don't forget to drink a lot of water.

16/8 Method

16/8 intermittent fasting means restricting food and calorie-containing drinks intake to eight hours each day and fasting during the remaining 16 hours. Many people choose to consume around noon and 8 p.m., so it helps them eat a nutritious lunch and dinner and a few snacks during the day while just fasting overnight and missing breakfast.

Others like to consume between the hours of 9 a.m. and 5 p.m., allowing enough time for a nutritious breakfast around 9 a.m., a regular lunch around midday, and a small early dinner or snack near 4 p.m. before beginning their fast. It can be done as often as you want, from once or twice a week to every day.

In recent years, 16/8 intermittent fasting has increased in popularity, particularly among those seeking to lose weight and burn fat. Some diets have stringent guidelines and regulations, but 16/8 intermittent fasting is simple to observe and yield actual results with little effort. As being less rigid and more adaptable than many other diet schemes, and it can comfortably fit into almost any lifestyle. 16/8 intermittent fasting is suggested to enhance blood sugar balance, cognitive activity, and lifespan and improve weight loss.

20:4 Method

The 20:4 method, a step up from the 14:10 and 16:8 approaches, is challenging to practice since it is very tough. This style of intermittent fasting is referred to as "intense" and "restrictive." Nonetheless, researchers say that the benefits of practicing this strategy are almost unrivaled to any other tactic.

For the 20:4 method, you can fast for 20 hours a day, bundle all of your dinners, eat, and snacking into four hours. People who follow the 20:4 diet consume two smaller meals or one main meal and a few treats during their four-hour feeding window, and it is up to them to decide which four hours of the day they dedicate to eating. The key to this approach is to avoid overeating or bingeing during those four hours of mealtime. If you are new to try this process, be cautious. Gradually work your way up to this one, and if you're already doing so, move to 20:4 when you're sure you're able to.

5:2 Method

This method allows individuals to consume an average amount of nutritious food for five days and then decrease their calorie consumption for the next two days. Women usually consume 500 calories over the two fasting days. These fasting days split during the week.

They can fast on Mondays and Thursdays and normally eat for the rest of the week. Between fasting days, there should be at least one non-fasting day. The 5:2 diet, also called the Fast diet, has undergone little research. A research on a sample of 107 overweight or obese participants highlighted that calorie restriction twice regularly, and constant calorie restriction resulted in weight loss. The diet also decreased insulin levels and increased insulin sensitivity in the patients, according to the report.

12: 12 Method

The diet's rules are simple and straightforward. Every day, a person must select and observe a 12-hour fasting window. According to several researchers, fasting for 10–16 hours cause the body to convert fat stores into energy, releasing ketones into the bloodstream. It will help you drop weight.

For beginners, this form of intermittent fasting strategy may be a flexible alternative. Because the fasting window is comparatively short, much of the fasting happens while sleeping, and the individual will eat the same number of calories per day. The most convenient approach to complete the 12-hour fast is to have sleep time in the fasting window.

An individual might, for example, fast between the hours of 7 p.m. and 7 a.m. They'd have to end dinner until 7 p.m. and wait before 7 a.m. to eat breakfast, but they'd be sleeping for most of the period in between.

24 Hour Water Fasting

Water fasting is a form of fast in which you don't eat or drink anything except water. In recent years, it has grown in popularity as an effective way to lose weight. Early in the morning is the perfect time to begin the water fast. Drink two glasses of water after getting out of bed. It is also helpful for bowel movements. At any point of the day, you can consume water. There are no restrictions to how much water you can consume at a time or how many times you can drink it. Go on doing this for the rest of the day until the following day. It can reduce the incidence of certain chronic diseases, lowers the risk of heart disease, certain cancers, and diabetes while also facilitating autophagy. It does come with a range of health risks and therefore is not suitable for all. Without medical observation, you shoundn't go on a water fast. Lime or orange juice is the perfect way to break one-day water quickly. Honey (half a spoon) can also be added to the juice. Fruits, which are simple to eat, may be taken if appropriate. Vegetables that boiled are often suitable to break the fast.

Eat-Stop-Eat Method

The Eat-Stop-Eat diet entails going without food for 24 hours for one to two days a week. Some people fast from one lunch to the next or from one breakfast to the next.

People on this eating plan can drink water, tea, and other calorie-free beverages during fasting time. On non-fasting days, people should resume their daily eating habits. This form of eating lowers a person's overall calorie consumption, thus keeping the individual's food preferences unrestricted. Fasting for 24 hours can be challenging, leading to nausea, headaches, and irritability. As the body changes to this new eating routine, many people feel that these symptoms become less intense with time.

Select a day when you are least physically productive to complete a 24-hour fast. Choose a day where you won't head to the gym or when you'll practice moderate yoga instead of a strenuous workout. It is an example of a strict schedule:

- Sunday: Consume 1,600-2,000 calories and engage in moderate exercise.
- Monday: Have lunch at noon and then fast for the rest of the day. Give yourself a day off from the gym.
- Tuesday: Skip breakfast, eat lunch, and then end your fast. Resuming physical exercise and eating dinner, as usual, is recommended.

Meal Skipping

Beginners can benefit from this flexible approach to intermittent fasting. It entails missing meals on occasion. People may select which feeds to cut depending on their hunger levels or time restrictions.

It is, however, important to consume nutritious foods at every meal. Individuals who track and respond to their bodies' hunger signals are more likely to succeed at meal skipping. People who follow this type of intermittent fasting feed when they are hungry and miss meals when they are not. For certain people, this may sound more comfortable than other fasting approaches.

Warrior Diet

The Warrior Diet is a form of intermittent fasting that is very intense. During a 20-hour fasting time, the Warrior Diet entails consuming very little, usually only a few portions of raw fruit and vegetables, and only enjoying one full meal at night. In most instances, the feeding time is just 4 hours long.

This form of intermittent fasting could be better for people who have already experienced other types of intermittent fasting. The Warrior Diet proponents contend that humans are regular nocturnal eaters and that feeding at night helps the body gain nutrients according to its circadian rhythms. People should make sure to eat lots of greens, proteins, and healthy fats over the 4-hour feeding period. Carbohydrates can also be used.

Although it is possible to consume certain items during the fasting phase, adhering to the rigid rules for what and when to eat in the long run can be difficult. Furthermore, some people find it daunting to consume such a big meal too close to bedtime. There's even a possibility that people on this diet won't receive enough nutrients like fiber. It will raise cancer incidence and have a detrimental influence on digestive and immune function.

Crescendo Method

Crescendo fasting is an excellent form of intermittent fasting for women since it is less demanding to their bodies. The simple approach is fasting for 12 – 16 hours twice or three times a week on alternating days. The "fasting window" for this form of fasting is 12-16 hours, and the "feeding window" is 8-12 hours. This type of fasting is a lot less challenging to follow. Simply skipping breakfast is a simple way to get started. Crescendo fasting for women is sure to result in weight loss. It is safer, less intrusive on a woman's hormones, sustainable, and less stressful on the body.

It will assist you in losing weight, reducing inflammation, and increasing your energy levels. On non-fasting days, higher impact exercises such as strength training or high-intensity intermittent training should be performed. During your fast, stay hydrated, drink plenty of water. You may also include drinking coffee or tea if no creamers, milk, or sugar.

Alternate Day Fasting

The alternate-day fasting plan, which includes fasting every other day, has many variants. Some people practice alternate-day fasting by excluding solid foods entirely on fasting days, while others accommodate up to 500 calories. People often want to consume as much as they wish on feeding days.

According to one study, alternate fasting is successful for weight loss and cardiac health in healthy and overweight women. Throughout the 12-week duration, the 32 participants lost 5.2 kilograms (kg), or just over 11 pounds (lb.).

Alternate-day fasting is a more severe type of intermittent fasting that may not be appropriate for beginners or people with delicate medical conditions. This method of fasting can even be challenging to sustain over time. Alternate-day intermittent fasting is entirely up to you, but it's an excellent place to start, particularly if you have a fluctuating schedule or are still getting used to one. The Alternate Approach could quickly become the Eat-Stop-Eat Method, Crescendo Method, or 5:2 Method if you choose to make it more extreme from this starting stage.

Chapter 4. WHAT TO EAT WHILE FASTING

What to Eat and Avoid on IF Diet?

IF is gaining momentum; perhaps the attraction arises from the absence of dietary restrictions. When you can eat is regulated, but what you can eat is not. That being said, what you consume too is relevant. Will you be breaking your fast with bottles of wine, frozen yogurt, and packages of cheese slices? Very likely not. So, let's have a peek at the best foods to incorporate into your IF diet.

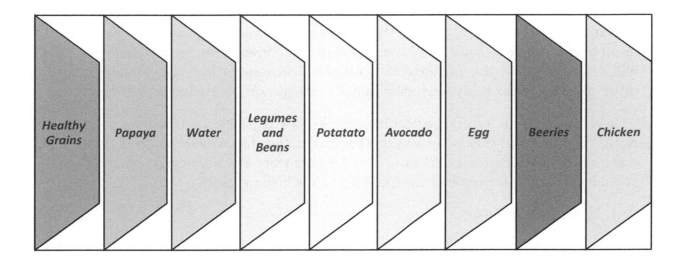

1. Healthy Grains

Carbs are a necessary aspect of life and are not the villain when it comes to losing weight. Since you'll be fasting for a significant portion of the day during this plan, it's vital to plan time for how you'll get enough calories without feeling bloated. While a balanced diet excludes refined foods, there is a place or time for the whole-wheat, breakfast sandwiches, and bread rolls, which absorb more efficiently and provide fast and simple energy. These can be a perfect fuel supply when out and about if you want to your daily workouts or practice daily during intermittent fasting.

2. Papaya

You'll probably start to feel hungry in the final moments of your fast, particularly if you're new to skipping meals. It can lead to you overeating in large amounts, making you exhausted and groggy moments later. Papain, a particular enzyme present in papaya, works on amino acids to break them down. Incorporating pieces of this sweet fruit into a high-protein meal will aid absorption and reduce bloating.

3. Water

Being hydrated is essential on any diet, but especially on an intermittent fasting diet. It is important not to get drained when fasting. Per day, you must consume at least eight cups of liquid. Make it a habit to drink the water each half an hour. You should also fill a 1-liter water bottle with water and leave it somewhere visible so that you are reminded to stay hydrated any time you glance at it. Many women experience pregnancy complications as a result of excessive water use. However, if you do not consume sufficient water, your fitness will deteriorate, and your digestive difficulties will worsen. Dehydration induces a slew of other concerns in the body, including jaundice, exhaustion, headaches, and dizziness.

If you can't drink water, consider fruit drinks, raw vegetables, coconut water, and other related liquids. Fruit shakes are also another choice, but they contain so many calories that one glass should suffice for the entire day. If you're using the 5:2 form of extended fasting, avoiding the smoothie is a smart choice because it's high in calories.

4. Legumes and Beans

Although many diets ignore legumes and beans entirely due to their high carbohydrate content, skipping breakfast allows you to indulge in a tub of legume and bean-packed chili periodically. Beans and grains are super helpful to your well-being. They are low in calories and leave you content for a lot longer. A balanced diet can have a variety of foods, and legumes are one of them. You should eat grains and beans a minimum of three days a week, if not more. It will also assist you in losing weight and establishing a healthy eating schedule. Consuming fast food is often significantly worse than consuming calorie-dense natural foods. Beans and legumes may be used in a range of dishes. While Cuban chili can come to mind first, grains and beans may be used in various other words, including curries, stews, sauces, and even roasting. Try frying chickpeas, lentils, or peas with pepper and salt if you're searching for lunch. In less than 10 minutes, you'll have a great tasting snack with no chemical flavors.

5. Potatoes

Unlike most diets, fasting has few carb limits or constraints. So, if potatoes are your thing, you're in fortune. According to health specialists, consuming potatoes throughout fasting is beneficial. Potatoes are the most excellent comfort food in every country, and because of their high value, they can be found all year long. It is also moderately priced and often regarded as among the most filling items. The human body quickly digests white potatoes. They're still a decent exercise snack when mixed with a source of protein to refresh the tired and hungry body. Another advantage of potatoes for the IF diet plan is that when they are cooled, they turn into complex carbohydrate that fuels healthy bacteria in the digestive tract.

6. Avocado

Avocado is one of those fruits that deserve to be listed on its own to highlight its importance! One avocado can sustain you working for at least 6 hours. There would be no hungry bouts or lightheadedness afterward. It's chock-full of all the positive stuff. It is, of course, one of the higher calorie foods, so you may question whether you should consume it as part of a weight-loss diet. However, a study has shown that it offers decent protein, which is essential for fat-burning. It helps you stay satisfied for a long time; this way, you're not overeating, which helps to lose weight. When the avocado is fully mature, it may be consumed on its own. You can create a feta cheese and avocado bowl with it, as well as guacamole, avocado smoothies, and tasty dips.

7. Egg

The egg is a nutrient-dense meal. The neurons need a certain amount of fat, which is present in eggs. An egg may be used in various ways, including breakfast, lunch, and dinner in the shape of egg curry. Eggs are necessary for baked goods, and if you like baking, using eggs in your standard meals is not a challenge. It will maintain you pumped up for at least 4 hours. Fasting may be taxing on the brain and mind, but getting superfood like an egg on hand is a safe idea.

8. Berries

Flavonoids are abundant in berries. They have a magical impact on health and hair. You will see how berries are often used in skincare items and advertisements. It is done purposefully: berries help to maintain the skin smooth and fresh. Berries such as blueberry, cherry, mulberry, mango, among others, are all helpful to one's well-being. They're also delicious. You don't have to think about calories if you consume half a cup of just about any berry a day. Berries also are tasty, but they can be consumed on their own. However, you can use them in savory dishes and pies, cookies, milkshakes, and juices. Cooked strawberries work as well.

9. Chicken

Skipping breakfast does not preclude all foods, and poultry is one that anyone likes and can handle adequately while on a diet. Tiny amounts of poultry can be used in your standard menu if you observe fasting. White meat is already thought to be beneficial to one's welfare. It does not trigger any of the health issues that processed meat may. In every region of the country, poultry and duck are readily available. Since turkey bird is not bred all over the world, you will need to do some research. Different forms of birds may also be served with a minimal serving amount. It's critical to monitor your meals whether you want to lose fat or enjoy a healthy lifestyle.

Foods to Avoid on Intermittent Fasting

Beginners sometimes make the error of consuming just about everything throughout their whole eating periods. They mistakenly think that all calorie intakes are equivalent and that the organs can burn the food they consume over the next abstinence period. Although your body will burn food you must always watch your diet to get the maximum performance throughout your fast.

The following foods must be stopped at all costs, but particularly during fasting diet feeding windows, when what you consume at that period directly affects your body and well-being. These foods can be avoided since they are high in calories and contain many starch, fat, and salt. They won't satisfy you after a short, and they might even leave you hungry. They often have so little nutrition.

1. Saturated and Trans Fats

Deep-fried products, artificial butter, and other butter substitutes, processed baked products, popcorn, candies, and a variety of other ready meals all contain trans-fats. This kind of fat is very unhealthy because it raises bad cholesterol, causes inflammation, and increases the risk of cardiovascular failure. Some foods, oils, and dairy goods include saturated fats. They are suitable in balance and are a strong choice for ketogenic diets and fasting. Although they cannot be eliminated, they should be consumed in moderation with optimal performance.

2. Preservatives and Sugary Foods

Fruit sugars are antioxidants that are good for you that have no adverse effects on your body. Refined sugars can be removed in sauces, desserts, frozen treats, candies, and other items. Monk fruit and xylitol are two sugar replacements that will please your sweet tooth while holding your blood glucose in control. Both are made from plant sources that do not involve sugar. Limit the following foods if you choose to stick to an intermittent diet plan:

- Sugar
- Barbecue sauce
- Fruit juice
- Cakes
- Ketchup
- Cereals
- Biscuits
- Popcorn heated in the microwave
- Sugary granola
- Potato chips

3. Excessive Amounts of Carb-Filled Foods

In limited to medium amounts, grains (buckwheat, rice, barley, wheat, and so on) may be a component of a balanced lifestyle. They have sustained energy and can be consumed before a long-distance athletic exercise, such as a sprint or riding, as a power source. Add rolled oats, sesame seeds, and other related seeds and nuts to reduce Greek yogurt or cereal grains.

Best Supplements for Intermittent Fasting

Despite the numerous possible advantages of fasting, it does have one drawback: nutrient loss. Fasting causes your body to lack the nutrition it usually gets from food, particularly if you exercise. The only way to compensate for this lack of nutrition is to consume high-nutrient meals at mealtime. Some individuals, though, do not get many nutrients and vitamins from eating. Supplements may help fasters fill nutrient shortages in this situation. Individuals who fast (or follow a time-restricted diet) daily will benefit from these supplements in particular.

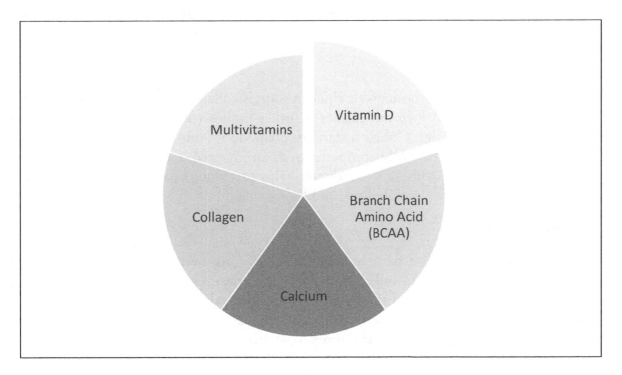

1. Vitamin D

Vitamin D deficiency is a regular occurrence. Fortunately, a quick blood examination will tell you whether you lack this immunity-increasing vitamin. Doctors still advise that you continue to reach your requirements by getting the sunlight every day. Some individuals, however, can need supplementation. Take the vitamin D with food in these situations because fat-soluble indicates the body requires fat to consume it properly.

2. Branch Chain Amino Acid (BCAA)

BCAAs (branched-chain amino acids) are a protein class (valine, isoleucine, and leucine). We can't create essential proteins on our own, so we need to get them from food. They're contained in important foods like poultry, beef, and dairy. Although this muscle-building supplement is best for those who love fasted cardio or intense exercises first thing in the morning, it may also be eaten during the day (fasting or not) to save the body from being catabolic and preserving lean muscle mass. BCAAs help protect musculature from disintegrating by encouraging our bodies to utilize energy from food for more extended periods, making them a vital substitute for skipping breakfast. Another benefit of BCAAs is that they tend to relieve muscle pain after an exercise.

3. Calcium

A regular calcium consumption of 1,000 mg is suggested for adults, approximately equal to 3 cups of milk. With a shorter eating time, consuming this much can be restricted, so high-calcium products should be prioritized. Vitamin D enhanced milk improves calcium intake and helps to maintain bone strength. You should add the milk to beverages or cereals, or consume it with meals, to increase your regular calcium intake. Non-dairy calcium options contain tofu and soy goods and also green vegetables like kale if you're not a lover of the shakes.

4. Collagen

One of the essential components of chicken soup is collagen. It may be obtained in fine powder and incorporated into milkshakes or other liquids to promote other soft tissues, lungs, tendons, and muscles. Collagen starts to break down into a more accessible form to digest and enhance specific body components when ingested. Collagen, like intermittent fasting, tends to increase muscle strength and helps to reduce bone loss. It's also good for the heart, brain, cognition, metabolism, and losing weight.

5. Multivitamins

One plausible explanation for why intermittent fasting causes fat loss is that the body will have less time to consume and consume fewer calories. Although the idea of fuel in and fuel out stands true, the possibility of vitamin deficiency while in a calorie deficit is seldom addressed. While a multivitamin isn't needed if you eat a well-balanced diet rich in fruits and veggies, living can get intense, and supplementation can fill the gaps.

Chapter 5. FOOD TO ENJOY/AVOID

Foods to Eat

- Eggs--Make sure you eat the yolk because this contains vitamins and protein!
- Leafy greens--We're talking about things like spinach, collards, kale, and Swiss chards, to name a few, and these are packed with fiber and low in calories too.
- Oily and fatty fish, such as salmon--Salmon is a fish that will keep you feeling full. Still, it's also high in omega-three fatty acids, which are ideal for boosting brain health, reducing inflammation, and generally helping with weight loss too. If salmon isn't your bag, try mackerel, trout, herring, and sardines instead.
- Cruciferous vegetables--In this case, you need to consider Brussels sprouts, broccoli, cabbage, and cauliflower. Again, these types of vegetables contain a high fiber amount which helps you feel fuller for longer, but also have cancer-fighting attributes
- Lean meats--Stick to beef and chicken for the best options but make sure that you go for the leanest cuts possible. You'll get a good protein boost here, but you can also make all manner of delicious dishes with both types of meat!
- Boiled potatoes--You might think that potatoes are rotten for you, and in most cases, they are, especially if you fry them. Still, boiled potatoes are a good choice, especially if you lack potassium. They are also very filling.
- Tuna--This is a different type of fish from the oily fish we mentioned earlier, and its low fat but high in protein. Go for tuna, which is canned, containing water and not oil, for the healthiest option. Pile it onto a jacket potato for a delicious and healthy meal!
- Beans and other legumes–These are the staple of any healthy diet and are super filling. We're talking about kidney beans, lentils, and black beans here, and they're high in fiber and protein.
- Cottage cheese–If you're a cheese fan, there's no reason to deny yourself, but most cheeses are pretty high in fat. In that case, why not opt for cottage cheese instead? It is high in protein and quite filling but low in calories.
- Avocados--The fad food of the moment is very healthy and great for boosting your brainpower! Mash it up on some toast for a great breakfast packed with potassium and plenty of fiber.
- Nuts--Instead of snacking on chocolate and crisps, why not snack on nuts? You'll get significant amounts of healthy fats, as well as fiber and protein, and they're filling too. Don't eat too many, however, as they can be high in calories if you overindulge.
- Whole grains--Everyone knows that whole grains are packed with fiber and therefore keep you fuller for longer, so this is the ideal choice for anyone who is trying intermittent fasting. Try quinoa, brown rice, and oats to get you started.

- Fruits--Not all fruits are healthy, but they're certainly a better option than chocolate and crisps! You'll also get a plethora of different vitamins and minerals, as well as a boost of antioxidants into your diet - ideal for your immune system.
- Seeds--Again, just like nuts, seeds make a great snack and can sprinkle them on many foods, such as yogurt and porridge. Try chia seeds for a high fiber treat while being low calorie at the same time.
- Coconut oil and extra virgin olive oil--You will no doubt have heard of the wonders of coconut oil, and this is a very healthy oil in cooking. Coconut oil is made up of medium-chain triglycerides, and while you might panic at the word triglycerides, these are the beneficial type! However, if you want to go for something deficient in calories, you can't beat extra virgin olive oil.
- Yogurt--Perfect for a gut health boost, yogurt is your friend because it will keep you full, and it also has probiotic content, provided you go for products that say 'live and active cultures on the pot. Avoid the overly sugary yogurt treats, and anything which says 'low fat' usually isn't as positive as it sounds!

Foods to Avoid

- Sugary foods may curb your appetite, but they won't do anything good for your body in the long run. Steer clear for your future ease.
- Highly GMO foods are also things to avoid when you're working through your fast. They can offset the actual nutrition being provided by other foods in your diet.
- Drinks to Take: you are allowed to take drinks while fasting. Go for drinks that are nutritious because they are suitable for the body. Some of the drinks that you can take are listed below;
- Water with fruit or veggie slices will provide nourishment and flavor for those times when you're fasting and need a little extra boost!
- Probiotic drinks like kombucha or kefir will work to heal your gut and tide you over till the next eating window.
- Black coffee will become your new best friend, but be sure not to add cream and sugar! They detract from the excellent work coffee can do for your body during IF.
- Teas of any kind are soothing and healing for various elements of the body, mind, and soul. Once again, be sure to omit the cream and sugar!
- Chilled or heated broths made from vegetables, bone, or animals can sustain one's energy during times of fast, too.
- Apple Cider Vinegar shots are great for the tummy and for healing overall! Hippocrates' remedy for any ailment included this and a healthy regimen of fasting occasionally, so you're sure to succeed with this trick.
- Water with salt can provide electrolytes, hydration, and brief sustenance for anyone whose stomachs won't stop grumbling.
- Fresh-pressed juices are always great for the body, mind, and soul, and in times of IF, they can sustain one's energy and mood during day-long fast periods, in particular.

- Wheatgrass shots are just as healthy as ACV shots, with a whole other subset of benefits. To awaken your body and give a jolt to your system, try these on for size.
- Coconut water is more hydrating than standard water, and it's full of additional nutrients, too! Try this alternative if you need some enhancement to your regular water.

Monitor & Assess Progress

If you are starting intermittent fasting to improve your health and lose weight, it is essential to take your initial weight, take measurements, and take pictures before you begin.

Scale Weigh-Ins

On the morning of day 1, it is vital to get on the scale either nude or in tiny clothes. It is important to weigh yourself before eating or drinking anything. Choose a time and entertain yourself. It will be known as your starting weight. It is crucial that you consider yourself and write this number down and enter it into your phone or an app that you are using to track your progress. I think you should write it down in a journal along the way to see your progress in real-time side by side.

It may also be a good idea to calculate your Body Mass Index (BMI) and your Body Fat Percentage; there are apps to calculate both. A simple google search can result in free calculators to get this information. To prevent my scale victories from being non-victories, I choose the same day and time to weigh myself, once a week, only once a week. While intermittent fasting, you will lose inches faster than you will lose pounds from the scale. You must understand that so that you don't get discouraged and quit. Therefore, I recommend weighing yourself and taking measurements and pictures to see what progress you have made.

Measurement Tracking

On the morning of day 1, it is essential to take your measurements. You will need to buy a measuring tape to have on hand. I purchased one in my favorite color to make me feel better about myself while taking the measurements. It is crucial to measure yourself before eating or drinking anything. Choose a time and measure yourself. These will be known as your starting measurements. It is essential that you measure yourself and write these numbers down or enter them into your phone or an app that you are using to keep track of your progress. I think you should write it down in a journal along the way to see your progress in real-time side by side.

I usually take the following measurements: neck circumference, waist, hips, arms, thigh, bust, belly pouch, and calf. You can measure more or less. I take three separate measurements from my waist and stomach area because I feel like three different body parts. I take measurements at the same time each day and week that I weigh myself.

Before & After

On the morning of day 1, it is essential to take pictures before, so you have proof of how you looked on day 1. It is necessary to take your photos before eating or drinking anything. Choose a time and get used to taking these pictures yourself, as someone may not always be around to help you with this (the same thing for your measurements, do this yourself). It will be known as you before picture.

I usually take pictures from all angles: front, back, both sides, one with a flexed muscle, etc. Whichever pictures you decide to take, do those same pictures each time you take pictures. My clothes fit to tell all of what is progressing and what is not or still needs work. Once I have my photos taken, I then use different apps to create collages to see the progress of the latest image with the newest snapshot. I spend hours studying every inch of my body on these pictures to make sure I see all my victories. It is the best way to track your weight loss progress.

Chapter 6. MISTAKES TO AVOID DURING FASTING

Now that you know all about intermittent fasting and how it should be done, you should also know the usual mistakes people make while doing the fast. These mistakes can prevent you from realizing the benefits and make the entire brief nothing but a complete waste. So, once you know what they are, make sure that you do not make the same mistakes yourself. If you do not want to make mistakes, the first and foremost thing you need to do is be aware of everything you are doing and know why you are doing them. It will ensure that you can quickly push yourself back on track, even if you are sometimes off the path. Also, stop beating yourself up for a cheat day or any mistake that you made. Just move on by accepting that it happened, and it cannot be undone. If you waste your energy in self-loathing, you will not be able to make plans.

Fasting Too Long Even at the Beginning

You must have heard me saying this plenty of times already; you need to take it slow. Do not rush the process. If you haven't tried intermittent fasting ever in your life, then you should start with a 48-hour fast or even a 24-hour fast, for that matter. Yes, you will have to lengthen the fasting window eventually, but that does not mean you have to do it now and at once. What you have to do is increase the fasting period but do it in small increments. If you do not follow what I said, it will be you who will be facing inevitable consequences, and they are bound to happen.

One of the first consequences that people have to face when they fast for more prolonged periods too quickly is that they become grumpy. They misbehave with coworkers and loved ones. And the worst part is that you might shove it away, saying that it's just your way of coping with fasting, but it is not. Also, due to your cranky mood, some people might even give you negative feedback, and in most cases, that is when people give up the fast and throw every effort down the gutter all at once. Tossing the whole idea out of the window because of such a situation is not worth it, and it would not have come to it only if you had increased your fasting period gradually.

The second consequence is that when people do longer fast, in the beginning, they cannot continue it after the first couple of days mainly because it becomes too unbearable for them. They feel tremendously hungry all the time. The process of intermittent fasting should not make you think jarred or stressed. Instead, it should be gradual and gentle. If you genuinely want to continue intermittent fasting for an extended period, you have to learn to make it well incorporated into your routine, and for that, you need to take it slow. When you start the longer fasts right from the beginning, you walk on the path of disappointment, and most people give up too quickly in such cases.

Not Eating the Right Foods

It is probably the biggest mistake that I see people have been making. If you have been trying to incorporate the process of intermittent fasting into your day-to-day life, then you also have to ensure that you are eating the right foods; otherwise, it won't work the way you want it. For starters, as you might know, fasting means that you have to learn how to get your appetite under control. And this means that you cannot simply grab that packet of chips or that bar of crunchy granola whenever you feel like it. There is a time for everything, and time is highly essential. But equally crucial is what you are eating in your eating window.

If you make the wrong choices, you will have a hard time controlling your appetite. When you rely on foods that are rich in carbohydrates, you will be deliberately making the entire process difficult for yourself; your need, along with your levels of blood glucose, is in a state of continuous fluctuation. When you are on a low diet in carbs, you will have more fats and proteins. It will increase your levels of satiety. In simpler words, you will remain full for a more extended period. Moreover, this will give your body flexibility in metabolism to tap into your fat reserves whenever your body is fasting and does not have enough glucose as fuel.

Also, some people use intermittent fasting as an excuse to eat whatever they want when they are in the eating window. That is not right and won't bring you any good results. You have to remember that this is not a magic pill, and nothing will happen on its own if you do not put in enough effort. Intermittent fasting indeed allows you to take your health into your own hands and maintain proper metabolism, but for that, your diet needs to be healthy too. You have to cut down on sugar and processed foods. You need to incorporate more and more whole foods that are rich in nutrients and low in carbs.

Consuming Too Many Calories

It is required to eat the right foods to get the nutrients you need. Please do not overdo it in the eating phase. When people fast, they have this idea that they have to replenish themselves by eating an equally heavy meal in the eating window. Never try to compensate for the time you were not eating. Sometimes people end up overeating to such an extent that they regret their actions and feel bloated.

Also, in case you have overeaten, please don't be too harsh on yourself because it will only make matters worse. Accept the fact because you cannot undo it in any way. What you have to do from now on is to prepare and plan your meals and keep healthy options in every meal. It will ensure that you don't have to think about what you want to eat when the eating window starts. A vital part of intermittent fasting is to figure out a balance in your routine where you can prepare healthy foods and not depend on processed foods.

Not Staying Consistent

It is probably true for everything on earth that it will not bring you results if you are not consistent with it. The same goes for intermittent fasting. But what is worse is that if you are not compatible, you will be stuck in a cycle where you make poor eating choices, and you will be so disappointed with everything that you will not feel like doing anything about it. That is exactly something you need to avoid, and for this, you have to be consistent. The best way is to follow a fasting regime that you can maintain for the long term. You need to understand that if you truly want to reap the benefits of intermittent fasting, then it also means that you have to do it for an extended period without giving up on it.

If you already feel that you will not stay consistent throughout the procedure, you need to sit down and figure out why. You need to find the reason behind it and then deal with it. Is it because you do not like the method that you have selected? If it is so, then try some other form. Or, is it because you're fasting and feeding window is wrong and you are having difficulty adjusting to it? In that case, you need to change the timings differently. Whatever it is, don't give up before figuring out the why.

Trying to Do Too Many Things at Once

It is also one of the reasons why people give up on intermittent fasting, especially beginners. There's an adage that says you shouldn't bite off more than you can chew. Suppose you are trying out intermittent fasting for the first time. You are also trying to maintain a daily gym schedule (which you don't usually do). On top of that, you are also trying to cook your meals (when you are habituated to take-outs). In that case, it is straightforward to feel stressed.

So, maybe you can start by training only three times a week and then you can help your family members in cooking your meals. If you do not have anyone living with you, you can skip the gym for now and maybe go for a run in the neighborhood in the initial days. Once you are okay with this routine, then you can incorporate the gym.

Now that you know the common mistakes, I hope this will help you to avoid them.

Chapter 7. WORKOUT AND INTERMITTENT

Strength training is significant for everybody, except after 50, it turns out to be more critical than any other time in recent memory. It stops being about huge biceps or ripped abs, yet instead, take on a tone of maintenance. For only 20 to 30 minutes per day, you can see considerable changes in your body's age. So how about we begin. The accompanying exercise will give you ten fantastic activities that ladies more than 50 can focus on during their workout.

A cardiovascular workout is best for the heart and lungs. It improves oxygen delivery to particular parts of your body, reduces stress, improves sleep, burns fat, and improves sex drive. A few of the more common cardio exercises are running, brisk strolling, and swimming. Within the exercise center, machines such as the elliptical, treadmill, and Stairmaster are utilized to assist with cardio.

Some people are satisfied and feel like they've done after 20 minutes on the treadmill, but if you need to continue to be strong and self-sufficient as you get older, you should consider including quality training in your workout. After 50, quality training for a lady is now not about getting six-pack abs, building biceps, or posturing muscles. Instead, it has changed to maintaining a sound, solid body and is less inclined to develop injury and sickness.

Squat to Chair

Seat squats are a beginner-friendly exercise extraordinary for building significant leg muscles like your quads, hamstrings, and glutes while offering the help of a firm surface.

1. Stand tall with your feet hip-distance apart. Your hips, knees, and toes should make all points forward. (Hold free weights in your hands to make it harder).
2. Curve your knees and expand your bum backward as though you will sit once again onto a seat. Ensure that you keep your knees behind your toes and your weight on your heels. Stand back up and repeat.

Forearm Plank

Although it's a challenge to do it correctly, the Forearm Plank fortifies the abs, legs, and core once you get command of it. It is also helpful in extending your feet' curves just as your calves, shoulders, and hamstrings.

1. On the floor with your lower arms level, ensuring that your elbows are adjusted straightforwardly under your shoulders.
2. Draw in your center and raise your body off the floor, keeping your lower arms on the floor and your body in an orderly fashion from head to feet. Keep your abs drawn in and do whatever it takes not to allow your hips to rise or drop. Rather

than 8 to 12 reps, hold for 30 seconds. If it hurts your lower back or turns out to be excessively troublesome, place your knees down on the ground.

Modified Push-Up

If you have trouble doing regular push-ups effectively, you can always switch to modified push-ups. It works on your upper body.

1. Start in a bowing situation on a tangle with hands beneath shoulders and knees behind hips, so the back is calculated and long.
2. Fold toes under, fix abs, and twist elbows to bring down the chest toward the floor. Keep your view before your fingertips, so your neck remains long.
3. Press chest rears up to the beginning position.

Bird Dog

It is a simple exercise that improves stability and reduces lower back pain. It also helps to maintain proper posture.

1. Kneel on the ground on all fours.
2. Stand at one arm long, draw in the abs, and stretch the opposite leg long behind you.
3. Repeat 8 to multiple times and then switch sides.

Shoulder Overhead Press

1. Start with feet hip-distance apart. Bring elbows out to the side, making a goal-line position with arms, hand weights are along the edge of the head, and abs are tight.
2. Press free weights gradually up until arms are straight. Slowly return to the initial point. Whenever wanted, you can likewise do this activity situated in a seat.

Chest Fly

1. Hold a couple of hand weights carefully shrouded and place your shoulder bones and head on top of the ball with the remainder of your body in a tabletop position.
2. The feet ought to be hip-distance apart. Raise free weights together straight over the chest, palms looking in. Gradually lower arms out to the side with a slight twist in your elbow until elbows are about chest level.

Standing Calf Raise

1. Remain on the edge of a stage.

2. Or then again, if you have a stage heart stimulating exercise stage, place two arrangements of risers under the stage.
3. Stand tall with your abs pulled in, the soles of your feet solidly planted on the progression, and your impact points looming over the edge.
4. Lean your hands against a wall or a solid object for balance.
5. Raise your heels a couple of crawls over the edge of the progression, so you're on your tiptoes.
6. Hold the situation briefly, and afterward, bring down your heels beneath the stage, feeling a stretch in your lower leg muscles.

Single-Leg Hamstring Bridge

1. Lie on your back with twisted knees hip-distance apart, and feet level
2. Crush glutes and lift hips off the tangle into a scaffold. Lower and lift the hips for 8-12 reps, then repeat on the opposite side.

Bent-Over Row

The composition is exceptionally significant with the twisted around the column, and the ideal approach to guarantee you don't get messy is to pick the perfect measure of weight. Slow, controlled developments are more incentive than snapping up an enormous weight and contorting everywhere in the shop.

1. When you have your hand weight stacked, remain with your feet shoulder-width apart. Twist your knees and lean forward from the midsection.
2. Your knees ought to be twisted. However, your back stays straight, with your neck by your spine. Get the bar with your hands (palms-down), only more extensive than shoulder-width apart, and let it hang with your arms straight.
3. Support your center and crush your shoulders together to push the load up until it contacts your sternum. At that point, gradually drop it back down once more. There's one rep. With a lightweight, go for four arrangements of eight to 10 agents.

Basic Abs

The best abs exercises are ones that work something other than one part of your muscular strength. Indeed, there are various layers of muscles (in addition to delicate tissue, nerves, and veins) that make up the entire stomach wall. Also, even though you can't see or truly feel them all, they're genuinely significant for keeping your whole body solid and stable.

There are various types of abs exercises. Here are two of them to keep it simple for you.

Abdominal Hold

1. Sit tall on the edge of a solid seat (or step with four risers) and spot your hands on the border with your fingers highlighting your knees.
2. Fix your abs and carry your toes 2 to 4 inches off the floor. Lift your butt off the seat.
3. Hold this situation; however long you can — focus on 5 to 10 seconds. Let yourself down and repeat. Proceed for 1 minute.

The Side Crunch

1. Bow on the floor and lean right over to your right side, putting your right palm on the floor. Keeping your weight adjusted, gradually broaden your left leg and point your toes. Place your left hand above your head, guiding your elbow to the roof.
2. Then, gradually lift your leg to hip height as you expand your arm over your leg, with your palm looking forward. Put your hand over while bringing the left half of your ribs to stay near your hip.
3. Lower to your beginning position and repeat 6 to multiple times. Complete two arrangements of 6 to 8 reps, and afterward switch sides.

Chapter 8. HOW TO PLAN AND GET STARTED

First, Make A Monthly Calendar

Mark the days you want to fast on a calendar, depending on the type of fast you've committed to. Start a record and end time on your fasting days so that you know what time you intend to begin and end your fast in the days leading up to it.

Please make a list of your days and cross them off as you go; this will keep you motivated and on track!

Document Your Findings

Keep a journal about your fasting journey. Take your measurements one or two days before the event. First thing in the morning, weigh yourself after you've used the restroom and before you eat breakfast. Also, do not weigh yourself while wearing heavy items, which may affect the scale's results.

Measure your height because it is related to your BMI (body mass index) score.

Take measurements around your hips and stomach; if you want, you can also take measures around your upper thighs and arms.

Please take a photo of yourself and include it in the journal as well; It reminds you of why you embarked on this journey in the first place.

Please make a note of everything you discover and keep a journal of it.

A journal is also a great place to express how you're feeling and, of course, what you're grateful for. A journal allows you to keep track of the physical aspects of your diet and the mental factors. Never doubt yourself; your journal should be a haven for you to congratulate and motivate yourself.

Make a Meal Plan

The simplest way to stick to any diet is to plan your meals; 500 calorie meals are typically simple and easy to prepare, but many other more complex recipes are available for those who want to spice things up. Who knows, maybe you'll come across a meal you'd like to eat outside of your fasting days.

Prepare your meals the day before your fast days; this helps you stay on track and reduces food waste

It is recommended that you keep your meal preparation and recipes simple at first, especially in the first few weeks, to avoid overcomplicating the entire process. It also allows you to become accustomed to counting calories and determining which foods keep you fuller versus those that leave you feeling hungrier sooner rather than later.

Make a note of your meal plan in your journal and on your calendar.

Reward Yourself

It is critical to reward yourself on days when you can resume normal eating. A small reward can go a long way toward reminding yourself and your brain that what you're doing is worthwhile and should be recognized.

A reward should satisfy one of our primal needs, which include:

- Self-actualization and safety.
- Social requirements
- Self-Esteem needs
- Food, water, air, clothing, and shelter are examples of physiological needs.
- Buy yourself a block of chocolate or a new piece of clothing to do anything that makes your heart happy!

Relieve Hunger

When you're hungry, you'll feel more uncomfortable at first, but these feelings will pass. If you do get a craving, drink some black tea or coffee to get you through the day. Coffee has been shown to reduce feelings of hunger; if you must add sweetener, do so at your discretion. You should be aware that some sweeteners can have the opposite effect and make you feel hungry.

Maintain A Busy Schedule

Keeping busy means that your mind does not have time to dwell on your current situation, especially if you reach for a snack bar or cookie.

It is also advisable to engage in some physical activity, even on fasting days. A 20-minute walk before the end of your fasting period will help you reach the final stages of the fast.

Practice Mindful Eating

As mentioned, we are inclined to eat for all sorts of reasons; happy, sad, it does not matter. The problem is that these feelings related to food become habitual, so we aren't, starving but because we feel good or even off, we seek to tuck into something delicious.

The art of mindfully eating is not to allow these habits to master your life. The concept is simple: teach yourself to look at something, for instance, a piece of cake, and think, "Do I need it or do I want it for other reasons?" You could decide to have a bite or two and leave the rest, but you may be less inclined to eat the whole slice (or whole cake) if you think mindfully about it.

The art of mindful eating is to revel in the food placed before you. Pay attention to colors, textures, and tastes. Savor each bite, even when eating an apple.

Your brain gradually begins to rewire itself when it comes to food and when it needs or wants something.

Practice mindful eating by:

- Pay attention to where your food comes from.
- Listen to what your body is telling you; stop eating when you are full.
- Only eat when your body signals you to do so, when your stomach growls or if you feel faint, or if your energy levels are low.
- Pay attention to what is both healthy and unhealthy for us.
- Consider the environmental impact our food choices make.
- Every time you take a bite of your meal, set your cutlery down.

Practice Portion Control

Controlling portion sizes can be difficult for most; society has also regulated us to what we think is the size of an average portion. We have access to supersizing meals too, which does not help those struggling in the weight department. In 1961, Americans consumed 2,880 calories per day; by 2017, they consumed 3,600 calories, which is a 34% increase and an unhealthy one at that.

To help you navigate how to portion your food better, consider trying the following: when dishing up your food, try the following trick. Half of your plate should consist of healthy fruits and vegetables, one quarter should be made up of your starches such as potatoes, rice, or pasta, and the remaining quarter should be made up of lean meats or seafood.

Alternatively, try the following:

- Dish up onto a smaller plate or into a smaller bowl.

- Say no to upsizing a meal if offered.
- Buy the smaller version of the product if available or divide the servings equally into packets.
- Eat half a meal at the restaurant and take the remaining half to enjoy the following day instead.
- Go to bed early; it will stop any after-dinner eating.

Get Tech Savvy

Modern-day society has plenty to offer us in terms of the apps we can use to help determine the steps we take. The calories we burn, the calories found in our foods, research, information, and motivation for lifestyle changes, especially diets and exercise. The list is endless. There are many apps on the market currently that can help you track your progress concerning fasting.

The best intermittent fasting apps currently (at the time of writing), and in no particular order, are:

- Zero
- Fast Habit
- Body Fast
- Fasting
- Vora
- Ate Food Diary
- Life Fasting Tracker

Make use of your mobile device to set reminders for yourself when to eat, what to eat, and when your fast days are. It works exceptionally well when using it to set reminders when you should drink water, particularly for those who find it hard to keep their fluids up.

Making the Change

Understand that intermittent fasting is not a diet; it is a lifestyle, an eating plan that you are in control of, and one that is easy to perfect. Before you know it, fasting will become second nature.

When to Start?

Begin today, not tomorrow or after a particular event or gathering. Once you have picked the fast that best suits you, begin with it immediately. Never hold off until a specific day; once you start, you will gain momentum, and it will become something that is part of your day, like many other things that fill up your day. No sweat there!

Measure Your Eating

Three days before you fast, it would be wise to begin to lessen the amount of food you are eating or dishing up less. It helps your body begin to get used to the idea that it doesn't need a whole bowl of food to get what it needs or feels complete.

Keep up Your Exercise Plan

If you have a pre-existing exercise regime, do not alter it anyway. Carry on the way you were before fasting. For example, take a five-minute walk, and the next day, change the time to 10 minutes of walking.

Stop, Start, Stop

Fast for hours, and then eat all your calories during a certain number of hours. Consider this as a training period.

Do Your Research

Read up everything about intermittent fasting this way; it will put to rest any uncertainties you might have and introduce you to new ways of getting through a fasting day. Check out recipes that won't make you feel like a rabbit having to chew on carrots all day if you are stuck with ideas of what to eat.

Have Fun

Lastly, have fun, and see what your body can do, even over 50. It is essential to know that just because you are a certain age doesn't mean you are incapable of pursuing a new lifestyle change. Reward yourself when it is due, track your progress, adjust where the need is, and get your beauty sleep. It is another secret to achieving overall wellness and happiness.

Know Your BMI

You can quickly determine your body mass index, or BMI, as it is more commonly known. In total, there are four categories that an individual can fall into based on this figure. That is underweight, healthy, overweight, and obese. The concept is simple: our BMI gives us quantifiable amounts when comparing our height with our fat, muscles, bones, and organs.

How to Calculate Your BMI

To calculate your BMI, equate your weight (lbs.) x 703 divided by your height (in).

Once you get your BMI, you can compare it to the body mass index chart to determine which category you are classed into.

Class	Your BMI Score
Underweight	Less than 18.5 points
Normal weight	18.5 – 24.9 points
Overweight	25 – 29.9 points
Class 1 - Obesity	30 – 34.9 points
Class 2 – Obesity	35 – 39.9 points
Class 3 – Extreme Obesity	40 + points

Chapter 9. TIPS FOR MOTIVATION AND SUCCESS

While Intermittent Fasting isn't tricky, starting a new diet is always a significant change.

Track Eating Behaviors

The reason that most diets fail is that most of them calculate a desired daily calorie deficit that is based on your initial weight. As you get slimmer, you require a smaller calorie deficit to lose weight. If you stick to the initial number, you are putting more strain on your body than it needs, so your metabolism slows down. Traditional diets are usually hard to maintain because you have to think about mealtimes and meal planning to make the diet unsustainable. Also, most diets don't address eating habits and particularly habitual and emotional eating.

Your weight gain could have a lot to do with your eating behaviors. Eating beside any other reason than being physically hungry is wrong. You could be eating out of boredom, stress or to compensate for unfulfilled emotional needs. The best way for you to determine why you are overeating is to track your meals, the reasons you thought you were hungry, and what you ate at that time. This approach will help you identify when, how much, and which foods you eat for the wrong reasons. It is easier for you to determine the nutrition you need when truly physically hungry.

Set Goals

A healthy weight loss goal is to lose between one and two pounds every week. If you start losing more, there's a chance that you are losing muscle mass. There's credible research to confirm that it's possible to lose lean muscle mass with Intermittent Fasting if you don't eat enough protein. You can be healthy when it comes to weight but still have high amounts of abdominal fat, which can cause many health risks. The goals with Intermittent Fasting depend on your health and weight goals. You can determine your diet goals by answering a couple of simple questions:

- Which improvements are you seeking? Do you want to:
  o Reduce the symptoms of illness,
  o Feel better,
  o Become more energized,
  o Lose weight, or
  o All of the above?
- Are you interested in practicing the diet long-term, or only until you meet your goals?
- How will you track the intake of macronutrients?

- What are your diet preferences?

Calculate Body Mass Index

Body Mass Index or BMI is an indicator of whether your current weight is healthy compared to your height. You can calculate your BMI by dividing your weight in kilograms by your squared height (m). If your results are between 18.5 and 24.9, you are healthy. Anything below 18.5 isn't beneficial. The ideal measure is 21 for women and 23 for men. However, this calculation doesn't account for body fat, waist circumference, eating habits, and lifestyle. All of this goes into how healthy you are.

Your BMI can be higher if you are masculine, which doesn't mean that you should lose weight if you are healthy. You can think of yourself as obese if your BMI is over 30. However, this isn't exclusive to the number because it's possible to have a healthy weight with unhealthy body fat. These are rough calculations that can cause you to think of Athletic and someone who is thinner but has more body fat as obese. However, calculating your BMI can help you determine your weight loss goals in collaboration with your doctor and a dietitian.

Calculate the Body Fat Percentage

Looking into your body-fat percentage will help you to understand what you should do to lose weight, for example:

- Which method of Intermittent Fasting is the most appropriate?
- Whether or not you want to incorporate the Keto diet in Intermittent Fasting?
- How much do you need to exercise, and what kind of exercises are necessary?

If you like exercising, Intermittent Fasting will help you lose body fat but preserve or gain muscle mass. As a result, you may not notice scaling down. However, even if you don't lose weight but gain muscle mass, you will still look slimmer.

To track how your body fat changes, you can use the body composition scales. These scales help you track how your muscle mass, your hydration, and your body fat change throughout your diet.

Calculate Waist-To-Hip Ratio

The waist-hip ratio or WHR is a more credible measurement because it accounts for your natural body shape. For women, an ideal measure is 0.8, while 0.9 is perfect for men. If your measurements are higher, you should work on your profile.

For calculating the WHR, you can use a tape measure and measure the circumference of the widest part of your hips and your natural waist, which is slightly above your belly button. After that, divide your waist measurement by your hip measurement.

Plan Your Portions

Calculate Basal Metabolic Rate

While measuring meals isn't required with Intermittent Fasting, it is desirable to maintain optimal health levels. To start, you should calculate your basal metabolic rate to find out how many calories you need to keep your weight and how many you need to lose it.

Calculate the Right Portion Sizes

When calculating portion sizes, keep in mind that 1 gram of nutrients translates to a different number of calories:

- Fat-9 calories,
- Protein- 4 calories, and
- Carbohydrate-4 calories.

Calculate the Daily Calorie Intake

In general, Intermittent Fasting doesn't require calorie restriction for weight loss. Still, weight loss and other health benefits of fasting will be more significant if you have a controlled daily calorie intake.

What to Expect

For most people starting with Intermittent Fasting, skipping breakfast is one of the most drastic changes. No matter how strange it might feel not to have breakfast, resist the temptation if the meal doesn't fit into your feeding window. Your appetite will be suppressed in the morning, and there's no use in eating if you're not hungry.

While most people don't experience severe hunger while fasting, it is possible to get occasional cravings. It happens because the majority of our eating is habitual. As a result of regular eating, the balance of the hormones in charge of hunger and satiety is disturbed. The longer you fast, the better will these hormones balance out. As you regain a healthy sense of your body's natural appetite, habitual cravings will decrease.

It's also not recommended to eat late in the evening, despite the intense cravings you might feel. Doing so will produce more significant amounts of insulin because insulin is maximally stimulated with eating at this time. If you make dinner your largest meal, you will slow down the weight loss. Your largest meal should be around 3 p.m., while the evening meal should be lighter.

What to Look For

You can choose between numerous Intermittent Fasting variations. Some of the ways to determine the right fasting plan are to consider the following:

- Do you need to eat in the morning, or can you delay your first meal?
- Do you get hungry in the evening?
- Do you feel like you want to fast on certain days, but not the others?

Answering these questions will help you determine whether you want to fast daily or fast a certain number of days during a week and eat as usual during the remainder of the week.

Intermittent Fasting Tricks to Make It Work

Here are some tips and tricks for ensuring that you have a successful fast:

- Drink plenty of water– as a woman; you should drink 1.5-2 liters per day. Make sure you drink water first thing in the morning.
- To keep your hunger at bay, drink coffee and tea as caffeine is a normal suppressant.
- Stay busy and do meaningful work. The more active you are, the lesser time you will think about food. Get out of your house wherever you can!
- Get your best work finished in the morning because you're going to be the most inspired and have a lot of energy.
- Keep it adjustable for you–the best way to do this is to fast at your speed, as the short suits your lifestyle, you're more likely to stick to it. Switch the diets around until you find the right one.
- For at least three weeks, please give it a good try-don't give up too quickly. It makes your body adapt to that amount of time.
- Use vitamins for your benefit.
- Try to delay the breakfast to see how long it can last. It can provide you with a clear example of the best times to fast and eat.
- Don't mention you're fasting to strangers–the fewer people you meet, the less' helpful thoughts' you're forced to hear. With you, you're doing this. Don't think about that.
- Don't forget to take advantage of training. Weight training helps build up your body, which in turn increases your metabolism.
- Protein is a friend of yours. When necessary, include it in each meal and also use vitamins to help you out.
- Eat well. Don't eat garbage on your non-fasting days. In the long run, this will discourage you. It is important to remember that the day's first meal will set the tone for the remainder of the day. Make it a good one!

10 Proven Tips for Managing Your Fast

Each segment will cover the practical tips that are needed to manage your days of fasting. If you continue with your intermittent fasting regime, these will benefit you.

1. When you get hungry, hunger suppressants help you get through the fasting window when you get thirsty. These include coffee, sugar, green tea, cinnamon, and chia seeds. Use these to help you get through!

2. The mixture of diet and exercise: This is possible; several tests have shown that it's okay! You're going to work out what time of day is better for your training after a while.

3. Getting tired or dizzy: This is usually due to dehydration, so make sure you're drinking plenty. Increasing your salt intake is also advisable–particularly if headaches become a concern.

4. I'm struggling here: The best way to avoid giving up is to stay busy. By getting out and doing something constructive, take your mind off food.

5. I'm too busy: This can be for your benefit because your focus will not always be on food. Prepare a quick that matches the current hours of work/commitments before this becomes troublesome. There's no reason for not doing that–particularly not that.

6. I'm going to gorge: Once you've accomplished your fast, assume that it never happened and continue as normal. When time goes by, this will make it easier, and the body will be adapted.

7. Things continue to crop up: That's why it's essential to prepare. Clearing your calendar with crucial things and adapting will be the same as how effective you are.

8. Meeting with the negativity: Not everyone knows the effects of fasting, so it's best to educate those who need to hear about it–relatives, close friends, etc. Others will try to put you off or freak you out, stopping you from setting off.

9. Maintaining the loss of weight: The fast is not a quick fix. It's a long-term change in lifestyle that will help you keep the slimmer/healthier image you love. It's also best to eat much better and keep this up all the way.

10. How to keep going: You need to relax if you feel tired. There is something the body is trying to tell you, and you need to listen. That is why it's recommended that you clear your schedule at the outset.

Chapter 10. MOST COMMON MISTAKES

When you are looking to make any significant adjustments in your life, it can take time to discover exactly how to do it in the best ways possible. Many people will make mistakes and have some setbacks as they seek to improve their health through intermittent fasting. Some of these are minor mistakes and can easily be overcome. In contrast, others may be dangerous and could cause severe repercussions if they are not caught in time.

Switching Too Fast

A significant number of people fail to comply with their new diets because they attempt to go too hard too fast. Trying to jump too quickly can result in you feeling too extreme of a departure from your routine. As a result, both psychologically and physically, you are put under a significant amount of stress from your new diet. It can lead to you feeling like the diet is not effective and like you are suffering more than you are benefiting from it.

It is not uncommon to want to jump off the deep end when making a lifestyle change. Often, we want to experience great results right away, and we are excited about the switch. However, after a few days, it can feel stressful. Because you didn't give your mind and body enough time to adapt to the changes, you ditch your new diet in favor of more comfortable things.

Fasting is something that should consistently be acclimated to over some time. There is no set period. It needs to be done based on what feels suitable for you and your body. If you are not properly listening to your body and needs, you will suffer in significant ways. Especially with diets like intermittent fasting, letting yourself adapt to the changes and listening to your body's needs can ensure that you are not neglecting your body in favor of strictly following someone else's guide on what to do.

Choosing the Wrong Plan for Your Lifestyle

It is not uncommon to forget the importance of picking a fasting cycle that fits your lifestyle and then fitting it in. Trying too fast to a process that does not fit your lifestyle will ultimately result in you feeling inconvenienced by your diet and struggling to maintain it.

Anytime you make a lifestyle change, such as with your diet, you need to consider your lifestyle. In an ideal world, you may be able to adapt everything to suit your dreamy needs completely. However, there are likely many aspects of your lifestyle in the real world that are not practical to adjust. Picking a diet that suits your lifestyle rather than choosing a lifestyle that suits your diet makes far more sense.

Taking the time to document your present eating habits before you embark on your intermittent fasting diet is a great way to begin. Focus on what you are already eating and how often and consider diets that will serve your lifestyle. It would help if you also thought about your activity levels and how much food you truly need at certain times of the day. For example, if you have a spin class every morning, fasting until noon might not be a good idea as you could end up hungry and exhausted after your course. Choosing the dieting pattern that fits your lifestyle will help you maintain your diet to continue receiving excellent results.

Eating Too Much or Not Enough

Focusing on what you are eating and how much you are eating is essential. It is one of the biggest reasons why a gradual and intentional transition can be helpful. If you are used to eating throughout the day, attempting to eat the same amount in a shorter window can be challenging. You may find yourself feeling stuffed and far too full of sustaining that amount of eating on a day-to-day basis. As a result, you may find yourself not eating enough.

You might also find yourself not eating enough. Attempting to eat the same amount you typically eat in 12-16 hours in just 8-12 hours can be challenging. It may not sound so drastic on paper, but you may not feel like eating if you are not hungry. As a result, you may feel compelled to skip meals. It can lead to you not getting enough calories and nutrition daily. In the end, you find yourself not eating enough and feeling unsatisfied during your fasting windows.

The best way to combat this is to begin practicing making calorie-dense foods before you start intermittent fasting. Learning what recipes, you can make and how much each meal needs to have to help you reach your goals is a great way to get yourself ready and show yourself what it truly takes to succeed. Then, begin gradually shortening you're eating window and giving yourself the time to work up to eating enough during those eating windows without overeating. You will find yourself feeling amazing at the end and not feeling unsatisfied or overeating as you maintain your diet.

Your Food Choices are Not Healthy Enough

Even if you are eating according to the keto diet or any other dietary style while intermittently fasting, it is not uncommon to find yourself eating the wrong food choices. Simply knowing what to eat and what to avoid is not enough. Spend some time getting to understand what specific vitamins and minerals you need to thrive. That way, you can eat a diet that is rich in these particular nutrients. Then, you can trust that your body has everything that it needs to thrive on your diet.

You must choose a diet that will help you maintain everything you need to function optimally. Ideally, it would be best to combine intermittent fasting with another diet such as keto, Mediterranean, or any other diet that supports you in eating healthfully. Following the guidelines of these healthier diets ensures that you are incorporating the proper nutrients into your diet to stay healthy.

Eating the proper nutrients is essential as it will support your body in healthy hormonal balance and bodily functions. It is how you can keep your organs functioning effectively so that everything works the way it should. As a result, you end up feeling healthier and experiencing more significant benefits from your diet. If you want to succeed with your intermittent fasting diet, focus on it.

You are Not Drinking Enough Fluids

When you are dehydrated, you can experience many unwanted symptoms that can make intermittent fasting a challenge. Increased headaches, muscle cramping, and increased hunger are all side effects of dehydration. A great way to combat dehydration is to make sure that you keep water nearby and sip it often. At least once every fifteen minutes to half an hour, it would be best if you had a good drink of water. It will ensure that you are getting plenty of freshwater into your system.

Other ways to maintain your hydration levels include drinking low-calorie sports drinks, bone broth, tea, and coffee. Essentially, drinking low-calorie beverages throughout the entire day can be extremely helpful in supporting your health. Ensure that you do not exceed your fasting calorie maximum, or you will stop gaining the benefits of fasting. As well, water should always be your first choice above any other drinks to maintain your hydration. However, including some of the others from time to time can support you and keep things interesting to stay hydrated but not bored.

The best way to tell that you are staying hydrated enough is to pay attention to how frequently you are peeing. If you are waiting in a healthy range of hydration, you should be peeing at least once every single hour. If you aren't, this means that you need to be drinking more water, even if you aren't experiencing any side effects of dehydration. Typically, if you have already begun experiencing side effects, then you have waited too long. You want to maintain healthy hydration without waiting for symptoms like headaches and muscle aches to inform you that it is time to start drinking more. It ensures that your body stays happy and healthy and does not cause unnecessary suffering or stress to your body throughout the day.

You Are Giving Up Too Quickly

Many people assume that eating the intermittent fasting diet means that they will see the benefits of their eating habits immediately. It is not the case. While intermittent fasting typically offers excellent results reasonably quickly, it does take some time for these results to begin appearing. How long it has taken you to transition, what and how you are eating during eating windows, and how much activity you are getting throughout the day contribute to your results.

You might feel compelled to quickly give up if you do not begin noticing your desired results right away, but trust that this will not help you. Some people require several weeks before they start seeing the benefits of their dieting. It does not mean that it is not working. It simply means that it has taken them some time to find the right balance to gain their desired results and stay healthy.

By tracking your food intake and exercise levels, you might find that you are not experiencing the results you desire because you are eating too much or not enough compared to the amount of energy you are spending each day. Then, you can efficiently work towards adjusting your diet to find a balance that supports you in getting everything you need and seeing the results you desire.

In most cases, intermittent fasting diets are not working because they are not being used correctly. Although the general requirements are somewhat the same, each of us has unique needs based on our lifestyles and fantastic makeup. If you are willing to invest time finding the right balance for yourself, you can guarantee that you can overcome this and experience great results from your fasting.

You are Getting Too Intense or Pushing It

Suppose you are focused on achieving your desired results. In that case, you might feel compelled to push your diet further than what is reasonable for you—for example, attempting to take on too intense of a fasting cycle or trying to do more than your body can reasonably handle. It is not uncommon for people to push themselves beyond reasonable measures to achieve their desired results. Unfortunately, this rarely results in them achieving what they set out to achieve. It can also have severe consequences.

Listen and pay attention to your body precisely what it needs is essential. You need to be taking care of yourself through proper nutrition and proper exercise levels. You also need to balance these two in a way that serves your body, rather than in a way that leads to you feeling sick and unwell. If you push your body too far, the negative consequences can be severe and long-lasting. In some cases, they may even be life-threatening.

Chapter 11. COOKING TIPS

Tips for a Fast Day Cooking

1. Increase the Amount of Low-Calorie

Green vegetables are difficult to eat and should be purchased a bit earlier if large quantities are needed. Stir-fried vegetables are delicious. It is best to steam lightly. Invest in a tiered bamboo steamer to promote health and cook protein and vegetables at various stages that are environmentally friendly.

2. Some Vegetables Will Benefit from Cooking, but Other Vegetables Should Be Eaten Raw

Cooking certain vegetables, such as carrots, spinach, mushrooms, asparagus, cabbage, and peppers, destroys cell structure without destroying vitamins, allowing them to absorb more food. Mandolin makes the preparation of raw vegetables quick and easy.

3. Fasting Days Should Be Low in Fat and Not Fat-Free

A teaspoon of olive oil can be used for cooking or sprinkled on vegetables to add flavor. Or use an edible oil spray to get a thin film. The plan includes fatty meats like pork. Add a light oil dressing to the salad. This means that you are more likely to ingest fat-soluble vitamins.

4. Lemon or Orange Dressing Acids Are Said to Absorb More Iron

That comes from lush greens such as spinach and kale. Watercress and orange are a great combination with a small number of sesame seeds and sunflower seeds or blanching almonds interspersed with a small amount of protein and crunch.

5. Cook in a Pan

The way to reduce high-calorie fats. If the food sticks, splash the water.

6. Dairy Products Are Also Included

Choose low-fat cheese and skim milk, avoid high-fat yogurt, and choose a low-fat alternative. Drop the latte and throw the butter on a simple day. These are calorie traps.

7. Similarly, Avoid Starchy White Carbohydrates

(Bread, potatoes, pasta) and instead choose low GI carbohydrates such as vegetables, legumes, and slow-burning cereals. Choose brown rice and quinoa. Use oatmeal for breakfast longer than regular grains.

8. Make Sure Your Fast Contains Fiber

Eat apples and pears, eat oats for breakfast, and add leafy vegetables.

9. If Possible, Add Flavors

Chili flakes kick a delicious dish. Balsamic vinegar gave acidity. We also add fresh herbs - they are practically calorie-free but give the plate its personality.

10. If You Eat Protein, You Stay Longer

Stick to low-fat proteins, including some nuts and legumes. Remove meat skins and fats before cooking.

11. Soup on a Hungry Day Can Be a Savior

Especially if you choose a light soup with leafy greens (Vietnamese Pho is ideal, but keep the noodles low), soup is a great way to consume the ingredients that you are fed up with and that you struggle with within the fridge.

Chapter 12. BREAKFAST RECIPES

SWISS CHARD OMELET

Cook Time: 5 mins | Servings: 2

Ingredients:
- 2 eggs, lightly beaten
- 1 tbsp almond butter
- 2 cups Swiss chard , sliced
- ½ tsp sunflower seeds
- Fresh pepper

Directions:
1. Mix the almond butter and Swiss chard and cook for 2 mins in a non-stick frying pan
1. Pour the eggs into the pan and gently stir them into the Swiss chard
2. Season with garlic sunflower seeds and pepper
3. Cook for 2 mins

Nutritional Info (Per Serving): Calories 260, Fat 21 g, Carbs 4 g, Protein 14 g

HEARTY PINEAPPLE OATMEAL

Cook Time: 10 mins | Servings: 5

Ingredients:
- 1 cup steel-cut oats
- 4 cup unsweetened almond milk
- 2 medium apples, sliced
- 1 tsp coconut oil
- 1 tsp cinnamon
- ¼ tsp nutmeg
- 2 tbsp maple syrup, unsweetened
- A drizzle of lemon juice

Directions:
1. Add listed Ingredients: to a cooking pan and mix well
1. Cook on very low flame for 8 hours/or on high flame for 4 hours
2. Gently stir
3. Add your desired toppings
4. Store in the fridge for later use

Nutritional Info (Per Serving): Calories 180, Fat 5 g, Carbs 31 g, Protein 5 g

SWEET POTATOES WITH COCONUT FLAKES

Cook Time: 10 mins | Servings: 5

Ingredients:
- 16 oz sweet potatoes
- 1 tbsp maple syrup
- ¼ cup fat-free coconut Greek yogurt
- 1/8 cup unsweetened toasted coconut flakes
- 1 chopped apple

Directions:

1. Preheat oven to 400 °F.
2. Place your potatoes on a baking sheet
3. Bake them for 45 - 60 mins or until soft.
4. Use a sharp knife to mark "X" on the potatoes and fluff pulp with a fork
5. Top with coconut flakes, chopped apple, Greek yogurt, and maple syrup

Nutritional Info (Per Serving): Calories 321, Fat 3 g, Carbs 70 g, Protein 7 g

BANANA SMOOTHIE

Cook Time: 5 mins | Servings: 1

Ingredients:
- 1 frozen banana
- ½ cup almond milk
- Vanilla extract.
- 2 tbsp Flax seed
- 1 tsp maple syrup
- 1 tbsp almond butter

Directions:

1. Add all your Ingredients: to a food processor or blender and run until smooth.
2. Pour the mixture into a glass and enjoy

Nutritional Info (Per Serving): Calories 376, Fat 19.4 g, Carbs 48.3 g, Protein 9.2 g

STRAWBERRY SMOOTHIE

Cook Time: 5 mins | Servings: 1

Ingredients:

- 1/2 cup 100% orange juice
- 1 large banana, peeled and sliced
- 1 cup fresh or frozen strawberries, thawed
- 1 cup low-fat vanilla yogurt
- 5 ice cubes

Directions:

1. Combine orange juice, banana, and half the strawberries into a blender container. Blend until smooth.
2. Add yogurt, remaining strawberries, and ice cubes. Blend until smooth. Serve immediately.

Nutritional Info (Per Serving): Calories 153, Carbs 32 g, Protein 5 g, Fat 1 g

SUMMER SMOOTHIE

Cook Time: 5 mins | Servings: 1

Ingredients:

- 1 cup yogurt, plain nonfat
- 6 medium strawberries
- 1 cup pineapple, crushed, canned in juice
- 1 medium banana
- 1 tsp vanilla extract
- 4 ice cubes

Directions:

1. Place all Ingredients: in a blender and purée until smooth.
2. Serve in a frosted glass.

Nutritional Info (Per Serving): Calories 121, Fat 1 g

PARADISE SMOOTHIE

Cook Time: 5 mins | Servings: 1

Ingredients:
- 1/2 cup 100% orange juice
- 2 /3 peeled peaches
- 1 cup low-fat vanilla yogurt
- 5 ice cubes

Directions:

1. Combine orange juice, peaches into a blender container. Blend until smooth. Add yogurt and ice cubes. Blend until smooth. Serve immediately.

Nutritional Info (Per Serving): Calories 123, Carbs 22 g, Protein 5 g, Fat 1 g

MELON SHAKE

Cook Time: 5 mins | Servings: 1

Ingredients:
- 2 cups chopped melon (cantaloupe, honeydew)
- 2 cups cold water

Directions:
Place all ingredients in a blender container. Blend until smooth.
Nutritional Info (Per Serving): Calories 27, Carbs 7 g, Protein 1 g, Fat 0 g

HEALTHY BAGELS

Cook Time: 5 mins | Servings: 8

Ingredients:
- 1 ½ cup warm water
- 1 ¼ cup bread flour
- 2 tbsp Honey
- 2 cup whole wheat flour
- 2 tsp Yeast
- 1 ½ tbsp Olive oil
- 1 tbsp vinegar
-

Directions:
1. In a bread machine, mix all Ingredients:, and then process on dough cycle.
1. Once done, create 8 pieces shaped like a flattened ball.
2. Make a hole in the center of each ball using your thumb then create a donut shape.
3. In a greased baking sheet, place donut-shaped dough then cover and let it rise about ½ hour.
4. Prepare about 2 inches of water to boil in a large pan.
5. In a boiling water, drop one at a time the bagels and boil for 1 minute, then turn them once.
6. Remove them and return to baking sheet and bake at 350oF for about 20 to 25 mins until golden brown.

Nutritional Info (Per Serving): Calories 228.1, Fat 3.7 g, Carbs 41.8 g, Protein 6.9 g

---

MORNING PUNCH

Cook Time: 5 mins | Servings: 6

Ingredients:
- 4 tbsps Lemon juice
- 2 cup peeled citrus fruits
- 1 cup ice
- 8 oz cranberry juice
- 1 ½ cup chopped pineapple

Directions:
- Place all ingredients in a food blender.
- Puree until smooth.
- Serve immediately.

Nutritional Info (Per Serving): Calories 116.6, Fat 0, Carbs 29.6 g, Protein 0

FRUITS BREAKFAST SALAD

Cook Time: 10 mins | Servings: 2

Ingredients:
- 1 cored and cubed Asian pear
- ½ tsp cinnamon powder
- 1 peeled and sliced banana
- 2 oz toasted pepitas
- ½ lime juice

Directions:
1. In a bowl, combine the banana using the pear, lime juice, cinnamon and pepitas, toss, divide between small plates and serve enjoying.

Nutritional Info (Per Serving): Calories 188, Fat 2 g, Carbs 5 g, Protein 7 g

MEDITERRANEAN TOAST

Cook Time: 10 mins | Servings: 6

Ingredients:
- 1 ½ tsp. reduced-fat crumbled feta
- 3 sliced Greek olives
- ¼ mashed avocado
- 1 slice good whole wheat bread
- 1 tbsp roasted red pepper hummus
- 1 sliced hardboiled egg
- 3 sliced cherry tomatoes

Directions:
1. First, toast the bread and top it with ¼ mashed avocado and 1 tablespoon hummus.
2. Add the cherry tomatoes, olives, hardboiled egg and feta.

Nutritional Info (Per Serving): Calories 333.7, Fat 17 g, Carbs 33.3 g, Protein 16.3 g

QUINOA BREAKFAST BARS

Cook Time: 2 hours | Servings: 6

Ingredients:
- 1/3 cup flaked coconut
- ½ tsp cinnamon powder
- 2 tbsp Coconut sugar
- 2 tbsp Unsweetened chocolate chips
- ½ cup fat-free peanut butter
- 1 tsp vanilla flavoring
- 1 cup quinoa flakes

Directions:
1. In a large bowl, combine the peanut butter with sugar, vanilla, cinnamon, quinoa, coconut and chocolate chips, stir well, spread about the bottom of the lined baking sheet, press well, cut in 6 bars, keep inside fridge for just two hours, divide between plates and serve.

Nutritional Info (Per Serving): Calories 182, Fat 4 g, Carbs 13 g, Protein 11 g

CHEESE & KALE OMELETTE

Cook Time: 10 mins | Servings: 6

Ingredients:
- 1/3 cup sliced scallions
- ¼ tsp pepper
- 1 diced red pepper
- ¾ cup non-fat milk
- 1 cup shredded sharp low-fat cheddar cheese
- 1 tsp olive oil
- 5 oz baby kale and spinach
- 12 eggs

Directions:
1. Preheat oven to 375 °F.
1. With olive oil, grease a glass casserole dish.
2. In a bowl, whisk well all Ingredients: except for cheese.
3. Pour egg mixture in prepared dish and bake for 35 mins.
4. Remove from oven and sprinkle cheese on top and broil for 5 mins.
5. Remove from oven and let it sit for 10 mins.
6. Cut up and enjoy.

Nutritional Info (Per Serving): Calories 198, Fat 11.0 g, Carbs 5.7 g, Protein 18.7 g

CHICKEN BREAKFAST BURRITOS

Cook Time: 5 mins | Servings: 2

Ingredients:
- 2 tbsp Italian salad dressing
- 1 whole wheat tortilla
- 1 sliced pear
- 4 oz cooked skinless chicken
- 1 cup fresh spinach

Directions:
1. Slice the chicken into small bite-sized pieces and arrange them on the tortilla.
1. Cover the meat with spinach and arrange the pear slices on top.
2. Drizzle with Italian salad dressing.
3. Wrap the tortilla around all the ingredients: until it's a snug burrito.

Nutritional Info (Per Serving): Calories 246, Fat 10.3 g, Carbs 23.6 g, Protein 15.6 g

---

CHIA SEEDS BREAKFAST MIX

Cook Time: 8 hours | Servings: 4

Ingredients:
- 1 tsp grated lemon zest
- 4 tbsp Chia seeds
- 1 cup blueberries
- 4 tbsp Coconut sugar
- 2 cup old-fashioned oats
- 3 cup coconut milk

Directions:
1. In a bowl, combine the oats with chia seeds, sugar, milk, lemon zest and blueberries, stir, and divide into cups whilst within the fridge for 8 hours.

Nutritional Info (Per Serving): Calories 283, Fat 12 g, Carbs 13 g, Protein 8 g

---

APPLE CINNAMON CRISP

Cook Time: 10 mins | Servings: 4

Ingredients:
- 1 tsp cinnamon
- 1 cup brown sugar
- 3 lbs Granny Smith apples
- 2 tbsp All-purpose flour
- 1 stick butter
- 1 cup oatmeal
- 1 tbsp granulated sugar

Directions:
1. Peel and core the apples, slice thinly.
1. Mix granulated sugar with flour and add the apples. Toss to coat.
2. Put apples into the bottom of a 5-6 quart crock pot.
3. Combine brown sugar with oatmeal and butter. Mix until mixture is crumbly.
4. Sprinkle oatmeal mixture on top of the apples.
5. Cook apples fully on high heat.

Nutritional Info (Per Serving): Calories 549, Fat 27 g, Carbs 71 g, Protein 6 g

Chapter 13. LUNCH RECIPES

CAESAR SALAD

Cook Time: 15 mins | Servings: 4

Ingredients:
- 2 chicken breasts, grilles
- 1 head romaine lettuce, chopped
- 2 cup grape tomatoes, halved
- Parmesan cheese strips

For the Dressing:
- 3 garlic clove, minced
- 1/2 lemon, juiced
- 1 1/2 tsp Dijon mustard
- 3/4 cup mayonnaise
- 1 1/2 tsp anchovy paste
- 1 tsp Worchestershire sauce

Directions:
1. Mix all the dressing ingredients in a bowl and whisk well to combine. Cover and refrigerate the salad dressing.
2. Mix grape tomatoes, romaine lettuce and cooked chicken in a bowl. Crumble the cheese crisps into smaller pieces. Add dressing on top.
3. Toss to combine and serve.

Nutritional Info (Per Serving): Calories 400; Fat 25 g; Saturated fat 12 g; Protein 33 g; Carbs 5 g; Fiber 4 g; Sugar 4 g.

THAI BEEF SALAD

Cook Time: 15 mins | Servings: 4

Ingredients:
- 1½ lb. flank steak
- 1 tbsp olive oil
- 1 tsp sea salt
- 1 cup cucumbers, chopped
- 1 head lettuce, chopped
- 1 cup grape tomatoes, halved
- ¼ cup basil, cut into ribbons
- ¼ cup cilantro, chopped
- ¼ cup red onion, sliced

- ¼ cup olive oil
- ¼ cup coconut aminos
- 1 tbsp fish sauce
- 2 tbsp lime juice
- 1 tbsp Thai red curry paste

Directions:
1. Mix oil, coconut aminos, fish sauce, lime juice, and curry paste in a bowl and whisk to combine.
2. Season steak with salt on all sides. Put steak slices in a single layer into a glass baking dish. Add half of the marinade over the steak.
3. Cover meat with plastic wrap and refrigerate for 8 hours. Cover the reserved dressing and refrigerate.
4. Mix lettuce, cucumbers, grape tomatoes, cilantro, red onion, and basil in a bowl. Cook beef in a hot pan until brown on all sides. Let beef rest for 5 mins. Slice against the grain.
5. Serve salad with beef and dressing.

Nutritional Info (Per Serving): Calories 426; Fat 26 g; Saturated fat 14.2 g; Protein 38 g; Carbs 7 g; Fiber 1 g; Sugar 2 g.

KALE AND BRUSSELS SPROUT SALAD

Cook Time: 15 mins | **Servings: 8**

Ingredients:
- ½ lb. Brussels sprouts, outer leaves and stems removed
- ½ bunch curly kale
- 6 slices cooked bacon
- ½ cup dried cranberries
- ½ cup walnuts
- 2 tbsps lemon juice
- ⅓ cup olive oil
- ½ tsp garlic powder
- 1 tbsp Dijon mustard
- ¼ tsp sea salt
- ¼ tsp black pepper

Directions:
1. Add Brussels sprouts to a blender and blend well until chopped.
2. Add kale leaves to it and pulse until shredded.
3. Whisk mustard, olive oil, lemon juice, garlic powder, salt, and pepper in a bowl until well mixed.
4. Add kale and Brussels sprouts and stir to combine. Add the cooked bacon, walnuts, and cranberries in it. Toss well. Serve.

Nutritional Info (Per Serving): Calories 192; Fat 17 g; Saturated fat 1.6 g; Protein 6 g; Carbs 4 g; Fiber 2 g; Sugar 3 g.

CABBAGE COCONUT SALAD

Cook Time: 5 mins | Servings: 4

Ingredients:
- ¼ cup of coconut oil
- ½ head white cabbage, shredded
- 1 lemon juice
- ⅓ cup dried coconut, unsweetened
- ¼ cup tamari sauce
- 3 tsp sesame seeds
- ½ tsp cumin

Directions:
1. Add all the ingredients to a bowl and toss well.
2. Cover and refrigerate for 1 hour. Serve.

Nutritional Info (Per Serving): Calories 309; Fat 5 g; Protein 12 g; Carbs 6 g; Fiber 6 g

GRILLED CHICKEN SALAD

Cook Time: 20 mins | Servings: 2

Ingredients:
- ½ lb chicken thigh, grilled and sliced
- 1 tsp fresh thyme
- 4 cups romaine lettuce, chopped
- 2 garlic cloves, crushed
- ¼ cup cherry tomatoes, chopped
- 3 tbsp extra virgin olive oil
- ½ cucumber thinly sliced
- 2 tbsp red wine vinegar
- ½ avocado, sliced
- 1 oz olives, pitted and sliced
- 1 oz Feta cheese

Directions:
1. Season chicken with a tsp of thyme, crushed garlic, pepper, and salt.
2. Preheat oil in a pan over medium heat. Cook chicken until golden brown.
3. Mix olives, sliced cucumber, chopped lettuce, sliced avocado, and ¼ cup tomatoes in a large bowl.
4. Add chicken to the salad. Sprinkle with crumbled cheese. Drizzle with olive oil and vinegar. Enjoy!

Nutritional Info (Per Serving): Calories 617; Fat 52 g; Saturated fat 4 g; Protein 30 g; Carbs 7 g; Fiber 4 g; Sugar 2.5 g.

ITALIAN SALAD

Cook Time: 15 mins | Servings: 4

Ingredients:
- 1 cup mixed Italian olives, pitted
- 6 oz. deli ham, diced
- 6 cups Romaine lettuce, shredded
- ¼ cup pickled banana peppers, sliced
- 2 medium Roma tomatoes, diced
- ¼ red onion, sliced

For the Vinaigrette:

- 1 tbsp red wine vinegar
- 1 tbsp Italian seasoning
- ½ cup olive oil
- A pinch of sea salt
- Black pepper, to taste

Directions:
1. Add all vinaigrette ingredients to a bowl and whisk well to combine.
2. Arrange all the salad ingredients in a large bowl and top with the dressing. Toss well to combine. Enjoy!

Nutritional Info (Per Serving): Calories 289; Fat 24 g; Saturated fat 7 g; Protein 11 g; Carbs 4 g; Fiber 3 g; Sugar 3 g.

GARLIC CHICKEN

Cook Time: 35 mins | Servings: 4

Ingredients:
- ¼ cup olive oil
- 2 crushed garlic cloves
- ¼ cup flaxseed meal
- ¼ cup Parmesan cheese
- ¼ tsp black pepper
- ¼ tsp paprika
- 4 boneless and skinless chicken breast

Directions:
1. The first step is to preheat the oven to a temperature of 425 °F.
2. Take a pan and add the olive oil to it. Sauté the garlic in the oil for about 2 minutes and then transfer that oil to a bowl.
3. Take another bowl and combine Parmesan cheese with the seasoned bread crumbs.
4. Sprinkle the black pepper and Paprika onto the chicken breasts and then dip in the garlic mixture and olive oil.
5. Now coat the breasts with bread crumb and cheese mixture. Make sure that the chicken is coated well on both sides.
6. Now place the chicken in a baking dish and bake for about thirty to thirty-five minutes.

Nutritional Info (Per Serving): Calories 156; Fat 14 g; Protein 1.5 g; Carbs 4.2 g

CHICKEN LEBANESE STYLE

Cook Time: 31 mins | Servings: 4

Ingredients:
- Juice of 1 lemon
- ¼ tsp. oregano
- 10 garlic cloves, crushed
- 2 Roma tomatoes cut into wedges
- 1 medium onion, cut into wedges and layers separated
- 8 chicken pieces
- 4 tbsps. olive oil

Directions:

1. In a large baking pan, drizzle 1 tbsp. oil and grease the pan.
2. Add chicken in one layer without overlapping any piece.
3. In between chicken pieces, add garlic, onions, and tomatoes.
4. Squeeze lemon juice evenly on chicken and drizzle with remaining oil.

5. Season with pepper, salt, and oregano.
6. Pop in a preheated 500oF broiler for 30 minutes.
7. Remove chicken and lower oven temperature to 350°F. Baste chicken with juices.
8. Return pan to oven and continue baking for 20-30 minutes more or until chicken juices run clear.
9. Now place the chicken in a baking dish and bake for about thirty to thirty-five minutes.

Nutritional Info (Per Serving): Calories 189; Fat 10 g; Protein 31.5 g; Carbs 6.9 g

TILAPIA LEMON FLAVOR

Cook Time: 30 mins | Servings: 4

Ingredients:
- 1 tsp. dried parsley flakes
- 1 clove garlic, finely chopped
- 1 tbsp. butter, melted
- 3 tbsps. fresh lemon juice
- 4 tilapia filets

Directions:
1. Grease a large baking dish with cooking spray and preheat oven to 375°F.
2. Wash tilapia filets under tap water and dry with a paper towel. Place on the greased baking tray.
3. Pour lemon juice and butter on top.
4. Season with pepper, parsley, and garlic.
5. Pop in the oven and bake for 30 minutes or until flaky.

Nutritional Info (Per Serving): Calories 157; Fat 10 g; Protein 23.5 g; Carbs 8.9 g

TACO SALAD

Cook Time: 40 mins | Servings: 4

Ingredients:
- 1 tablespoon chili powder
- 1 teaspoon ground cumin
- ½ teaspoon onion powder
- ½ teaspoon garlic powder
- 1 pound lean ground beef
- ¾ cup of water
- 6 cups shredded Romaine lettuce
- 4 tablespoons taco sauce
- 4 ounces medium jicama (Mexican turnip), cut into thin strips
- 1 cup shredded fat-free Monterey Jack cheese

- ½ cup shredded fat-free cheddar cheese
- 4 tablespoons fat-free sour cream

Directions:
1. Make the seasoning mix: In a small bowl, combine the chili powder, cumin, onion powder, and garlic powder. Set aside.
2. In a large skillet, cook the ground beef over medium heat until browned, about 15 minutes.
3. Drain off fat, if any. Add the water and seasoning mix; stir to combine. Reduce heat to medium-low, and cook until liquid is almost completely absorbed 10 to 12 minutes.
4. In a large bowl, toss lettuce with taco sauce. Divide among four large serving bowls, about 1 ½ cups each. Top each with ¼ cup chopped jicama.
5. In a medium bowl, toss the Monterey jack and cheddar cheeses together; divide and sprinkle over the jicama.
6. Spoon the beef mixture (about ½ cup per serving) over the cheese.
7. Top each with one tablespoon sour cream.
8. Serve!

Nutritional Info (Per Serving): Calories 293; Fat 4.8 g; Protein 37.5 g; Carbs 11.9 g; Fiber 2.8g

SHRIMP GUMBO

Cook Time: 40 mins | Servings: 4

Ingredients:
- 3 tablespoons extra virgin olive oil, divided
- 2 tablespoons gluten-free All-Purpose Low-Carb Baking Mix
- 2 celery stalks, chopped
- 1 small green bell pepper, seeded and chopped
- 1 small onion, chopped
- 5 ½ cups chicken broth
- 1 cup diced stewed tomatoes
- 2 teaspoons Creole seasoning blend
- 2 tablespoons garlic cloves, chopped
- 1 pound collard greens, washed, cut in strips, or two packages (10-ounces each) frozen
- 1 (10-ounce) package frozen cut okra
- 2 pounds large shrimp, shelled and deveined

Directions:
1. In a large saucepan, heat oil over medium heat, whisk in baking mix, and cook, whisking, until deep golden brown, about five minutes.
2. Add celery, bell pepper, and onion and cook 5 minutes, occasionally stirring, five minutes. Add garlic and creole seasoning and cook for one minute longer.

3. Add chicken broth and tomatoes to vegetable mixture and bring to a boil. Add collards and okra, cover, and cook until collards are tender, about five minutes.
4. Add shrimp to gumbo, mix well, cover, and cook four minutes, until shrimp are pink and cooked through.
5. Season to taste with hot pepper sauce, salt, and pepper.

Nutritional Info (Per Serving): Calories 279; Fat 81 g; Protein 36.5 g; Carbs 18.9 g

ROST BEEF AND MIXED GREENS

Cook Time: 25 mins | Servings: 4

Ingredients:
- 48 ounces lean roast beef
- 8 cups mixed greens
- 16 ounces pickled okra
- 40 radishes, sliced

Directions:
1. Season roast beef with salt and freshly ground pepper.
2. Slice or cut the beef into cubes, and serve cold or slightly warmed in the microwave.
3. Toss greens, okra, and radishes with dressing. Serve salad with roast beef.

Nutritional Info (Per Serving): Calories 385; Fat 44 g; Protein 44.8 g; Carbs 38.9

INDIAN CHICKEN CURRY

Cook Time: 18 mins | Servings: 6

Ingredients:
- 3 tbsp. unsalted butter
- 2 garlic cloves, minced
- 4 chicken breasts, boneless, skinless
- 1 tsp. cumin
- ½ tsp. coriander
- ½ tsp. ground ginger
- ¼ tsp. crushed red pepper flakes
- ½ cup chicken broth
- ⅓ cup heavy cream

Directions:
1. In a large skillet, melt the butter. Sauté the garlic for 2 minutes.
2. Add the chicken breasts. Cook thoroughly.

3. Once cooked, remove the chicken and cut it into chunks. Return to the pan.
4. Pour in the chicken broth, cumin, coriander, ginger, red pepper flakes.
5. Turn down the heat to medium-low. Simmer 5 minutes.
6. Stir in the cream. Simmer another 3 minutes.

Nutritional Info (Per Serving): Calories 413; Fat 22 g; Protein 49.8 g; Carbs 4.9 g

BAKED BRIE

Cook Time: 12 mins | Servings: 6

Ingredients:
- 8 oz. Brie wheel cheese
- ¼ cup pine nuts

Directions:
1. Heat oven to 450°F
2. Trip top of white rind off the cheese.
3. Cover top with pine nuts.
4. Place cheese on aluminum foil pan or pie dish.
5. Bake 10 minutes. Serve.

Nutritional Info (Per Serving): Calories 144; Fat 12 g; Protein 9.8 g; Carbs 2.9 g

PORK MEATBALLS

Cook Time: 10 mins | Servings: 4

Ingredients:
- 2 tbsp avocado oil
- 1 tbsp chopped cilantro
- 3 tbsp almond flour
- 2 whisked egg
- 10 oz. no-salt-added canned tomato sauce
- Black pepper
- 2 lbs. ground pork

Directions:
1. In a bowl, combine the pork with the flour and the other Ingredients: except the sauce and the oil, stir well and shape medium meatballs out of this mix.
2. Heat up a pan with the oil over medium heat, add the meatballs and brown for 3 mins on each side.
3. Add the sauce, toss gently, bring to a simmer and cook over medium heat for 20 mins more.

4. Divide everything into bowls and serve.

Nutritional Info (Per Serving): Calories 332; Fat 18 g; Protein 25.8 g; Carbs 12.9 g

---

SHRIMP PASTA PRIMAVERA

Cook Time: 15 mins | Servings: 2

Ingredients:
- 2 tbsp olive oil
- 1 tbsp garlic, minced
- 2 cups assorted fresh vegetables, chopped coarsely (zucchini, broccoli, asparagus or whatever you prefer)
- 4 oz frozen shrimp, cooked, peeled, and deveined
- Freshly ground black pepper
- Juice of ½ lemon
- 4 oz whole-wheat angel-hair pasta, cooked per package instructions
- 2 tbsp grated Parmesan cheese

Directions:
1. Heat the oil in a large nonstick skillet over medium heat. Add the garlic and sauté for 1 minute.
2. Add vegetables and sauté until crisp tender (about 3 to 4 mins)
3. Add the shrimp and sauté until just heated through. Season lightly with salt and pepper and squeeze lemon juice over the shrimp and vegetables. Continue to cook for about 2 mins until the juices have been reduced by about half. Remove from heat
4. Toss shrimp and vegetables with pasta. Serve topped with Parmesan cheese

Nutritional Info (Per Serving): Calories 439; Fat 16 g; Protein 23 g; Carbs 50 g

---

SALMON AND POTATOES MIX

Cook Time: 5 mins | Servings: 4

Ingredients:
- 4 oz. chopped smoked salmon
- 1 tbsp essential olive oil
- Black pepper
- 1 tbsp chopped chives
- ¼ cup coconut cream
- 1 ½ lbs. chopped potatoes
- 2 tsps. Prepared horseradish

Directions:

1. Heat up a pan using the oil over medium heat, add potatoes and cook for 10 mins.
2. Add salmon, chives, horseradish, cream and black pepper, toss, cook for 1 minute more, divide between plates and serve.

Nutritional Info (Per Serving): Calories 233; Fat 6 g; Protein 11 g; Carbs 9 g

Chapter 14. DINNER RECIPES

BALSAMIC CHICKEN WITH VEGETABLES

Cook Time: 30 mins | Servings: 4

Ingredients:

- 10 asparaguses, ends trimmed and cut in half
- 8 boneless, skinless chicken thighs, fat trimmed
- 2 bell peppers, sliced into strips
- ½ cup carrots, cut into 3-inch pieces
- 1 red onion, chopped into large chunks
- ¼ cup + 1 tbsp balsamic vinegar
- 5 oz. mushrooms, sliced
- 2 tbsp olive oil
- ½ tbsp dried oregano
- 2 sage leaves, chopped
- 2 garlic cloves, smashed and chopped
- 1 tsp salt and pepper, to taste
- Cooking spray

Directions:

1. Preheat the oven to 425°F.
2. Season chicken with salt and pepper and spray 2 large baking sheets with cooking spray.
3. Mix all the ingredients in a bowl and mix well. Place everything on the prepared baking sheet and spread it in a single layer.
4. Bake for 25 mins. Serve.

Nutritional Info (Per Serving): Calories 450; Fat 17 g; Saturated fat 3 g; Protein 48 g; Carbs 4 g; Fiber 11 g; Sugar 2 g.

LOW CARB CHILI

Cook Time: 40 mins | Servings: 6

Ingredients:

- 1 bell pepper, chopped
- 1¼ lb. ground beef
- 8 oz. tomato paste
- 1½ tomato, chopped

- 2 celery sticks, chopped
- ½ cup onion, chopped
- 1½ tsp cumin
- ¾ cup of water
- 1½ tsp chili powder
- 1½ tsp salt & pepper

Directions:

1. Cook the meat in a frying pan until brown. Drain the excess fat and season meat with salt.
2. Add peppers and onions to the pan and cook for 2 mins. Mix onions, cooked meat, peppers, tomatoes, water, celery, and tomato paste in a pot.
3. Add the spices to the pot. Bring to a boil and reduce the heat to low-medium. Cook for 2 hours while stirring every 30 mins. Serve.

Nutritional Info (Per Serving): Calories 348; Fat 28.8 g; Saturated fat 8.5 g; Protein 14.9 g; Carbs 5.2 g; Fiber 2 g; Sugar 3.3 g.

CHEESY TUNA PASTA

Cook Time: 25 mins | Servings: 4

Ingredients:

- 4 cups zucchini noodles, spiralized, cooked
- 1 cup cheddar, grated
- 1 cup yellowfin tuna in olive oil
- 7 oz. basil pesto
- 1½ cup punnet cherry tomato halved

Directions:

1. Mix pesto and tuna with oil in a bowl. Mash well. Add in ⅓ of the cheese and add all the tomatoes.
2. Add noodles to the bowl, toss well to coat. Transfer the mixture to a baking dish and add the remaining cheese on top.
3. Broil the dish for 4 mins. Serve.

Nutritional Info (Per Serving): Calories 696; Fat 27 g; Saturated fat 11 g; Protein 40 g; Carbs 10 g; Fiber 4 g; Sugar 5 g.

SALMON WITH CAULIFLOWER RICE

Cook Time: 40 mins | **Servings:** 3

Ingredients:

- 1 tbsp olive oil
- 3 salmon fillets
- 1 tbsp coconut aminos
- 1 tsp fish sauce
- 1 tbsp butter
- 3 garlic cloves
- 1 cup basil leaves, chopped
- ¼ cup hemp hearts
- ½ cup olive oil
- 1 lemon juice
- ½ tsp pink salt
- 3 cups riced cauliflower, frozen
- 1 scoop MCT Powder
- Pinch salt

Directions:

1. Add fish sauce, coconut aminos, and olive oil to a baking dish. Pat the salmon fillets dry and add place into the dish skin side down. Add a pinch of salt. Let rest for 20 mins.
2. Heat an iron skillet on medium heat.
3. Peel and dice the garlic and add it to a blender. Add hemp hearts, basil, lemon juice, olive oil, MCT powder, and salt. Pulse well to combine.
4. Heat cauliflower rice in a skillet. Add pesto and pink salt. Mix well to combine. Lower the heat and keep it warm.
5. Add butter to the iron skillet placed over medium heat. Add salmon skin side down. Cook for 5 mins. Flip the salmon and add the remaining marinade from the plate. Sear for 2 mins.
6. Remove from heat and serve on top of rice. Enjoy!

Nutritional Info (Per Serving): Calories 647; Fat 51 g; Saturated fat 10.8 g; Protein 33.8 g; Carbs 5 g; Fiber 3 g; Sugar 3 g.

MUSHROOM BACON SKILLET

Cook Time: 10 mins | **Servings:** 1

Ingredients:

- ½ tsp salt
- 1 tbsp garlic, minced
- 4 slices pastured pork bacon, cut into ½-inch pieces

- 2 sprigs thyme, leaves only
- 2 cups mushrooms, halved

Directions:

1. Preheat a skillet over medium heat. Add bacon and cook until crispy. Remove from the pan.
2. Add sliced mushrooms. Saute until soft, stirring often.
3. Add garlic, thyme, and salt. Cook for 5 mins more, stirring often.
4. When mushrooms become golden, turn the heat off.
5. Garnish mushroom bacon with greens and enjoy!

Nutritional Info (Per Serving): Calories 313; Fat 8.5 g; Saturated fat 3.8 g; Protein 13.6 g; Carbs 0.3 g; Fiber 8.1 g; Sugar 2.2 g.

CHICKEN PARMESAN

Cook Time: 19 mins | Servings: 8

Ingredients:

- 2 lbs boneless skinless chicken breast
- 4 oz mozzarella
- ½ cup sugar-free marinara
- 1 cup almond flour
- 1 cup parmesan cheese grated
- 2 eggs
- 1 tsp Italian seasoning
- ½ tsp black pepper
- ½ tsp sea salt

Directions:

1. Add chicken to a plastic bag and pound until about ½-inch thick.
2. Add 1 tsp Italian seasoning, a cup of parmesan cheese, ½ tsp sea salt, a cup of almond flour, and ½ tsp pepper. Mix well.
3. Add eggs to a separate bowl and whisk well. Pat dry the chicken with paper towels.
4. Dip chicken into the egg mixture and then coat with almond flour mixture. Brush with oil or coat with cooking spray.
5. Preheat the oven to 425°F. Place chicken on a baking sheet lined with parchment paper. Cook for about 11-12 mins.
6. Then flip the chicken, spray with cooking spray and cook for 5 mins more.
7. Sprinkle each piece with mozzarella and drizzle with pasta sauce. Transfer back to the oven and cook for a few mins until cheese is melted.

Nutritional Info (Per Serving): Calories 318; Fat 17 g; Saturated fat 5 g; Protein 36 g; Carbs 3 g; Fiber 1 g; Sugar 1 g

SHRIMP CURRY

Cook Time: 8 mins | Servings: 5

Ingredients:

- 1 tsp. garam masala
- ¼ cup of water
- 2 lbs. medium shrimp, peeled and deveined
- 1 tsp. ground red Chile pepper
- 1 tomato, finely chopped
- ½ tsp. ground turmeric
- 2/3 tsp. salt
- 1 tsp. ground coriander
- 1 tbsp. ginger garlic paste
- 10 fresh curry leaves
- 1 large onion, chopped
- ¼ cup of vegetable oil

Directions:

1. On high fire, place a large saucepan and heat oil.
2. Sauté onions for 3-5 minutes or until lightly browned.
3. Add salt, coriander, ginger-garlic paste, and curry leaves. Fry for a minute.
4. Add water, shrimp, Chile powder, tomato, salt, and turmeric.
5. Lower fire to medium-high and continue sautéing shrimps until cooked, around 7 to 8 minutes
6. Season with garam masala, sauté for a minute, and turn off the fire.

Nutritional Info (Per Serving): Calories 211; Fat 11 g; Protein 30 g; Carbs 5 g; Fiber 1.5 g

SALMON WITH BASIL TOMATO

Cook Time: 20 mins | Servings: 2

Ingredients:

- 2 tbsps. grated Parmesan cheese
- 1 tbsp. olive oil
- 1 tomato, sliced thinly

- 1 tbsp. dried basil
- 2 6-oz boneless salmon fillet
- Pepper and salt to taste

Directions:

1. Line a baking sheet with aluminum foil, grease with cooking spray, and preheat the oven to 375°F.
2. Place salmon on greased foil with skin side down.
3. Sprinkle with basil, top salmon with tomato slices, and season with pepper, salt, Olive oil, and Parmesan cheese.
4. Pop in the oven and bake for 20 minutes or until Parmesan cheese is lightly browned.

Nutritional Info (Per Serving): Calories 191; Fat 13 g; Protein 35 g; Carbs 8 g; Fiber 1.8 g

LEMON BROCCOLI SOUP

Cook Time: 11 mins | Servings: 2

Ingredients:

- to 3 - lbs. of fresh broccoli florets
- 4 cups of water
- 2 cups unsweetened almond milk
- ¾ cup parmesan cheese
- 2 tbsp. lemon juice

Directions:

1. Put the broccoli and water in a substantial pan. Spread and cook on medium-high until the broccoli is delicate.
2. Save one measure of the cooling fluid and dispose of the rest.
3. Include half of the broccoli, the saved cooking fluid, and almond milk into a blender. Mix until smooth.
4. Come back to the pot with whatever is left of the broccoli. Include the parmesan and lemon squeeze and warmth until hot.
5. I didn't include salt or pepper; however, you might need to have a bit. Simply season to taste.

Nutritional Info (Per Serving): Calories 371; Fat 11 g; Protein 15 g; Carbs 9 g; Fiber 1.9 g

CHICKEN WINGS

Cook Time: 30 mins | Servings: 6

Ingredients:

- ½ serving all-purpose low carb baking mix
- 2 Tbsp. chili powder
- 1 tsp. cayenne pepper
- 2 tsp. yellow mustard seed
- 2 tsp. salt
- 12-16 chicken wings

Directions:

1. Preheat oven to 450°F
2. Rinse the chicken wings.
3. Line a baking sheet with aluminum foil. Spray with non-stick cooking spray.
4. Take a Ziploc bag; add the baking mix, chili powder, cayenne pepper, and mustard seed, salt. Place the wings in the bag. Massage the chicken wings through the pack to coat them with seasoning.
5. Transfer to the baking sheet. Cook 30-35 minutes, until golden brown.
6. Serve immediately.

Nutritional Info (Per Serving): Calories 271; Fat 18 g; Protein 22 g; Carbs 9 g; Fiber0.9 g

TACO CASSEROLE RECIPE

Cook Time: 22 mins | Servings: 6

Ingredients:

- 2 lb. ground turkey or beef
- 2 tbsp. taco seasoning
- 1 cup salsa
- 16 oz. cottage cheese
- 8 oz. shredded cheddar cheese

Directions:

1. Preheat stove to 400°F.
2. Blend the ground meat and taco flavoring in a vast meal dish. Mine is 11 x 13. Prepare for 20 minutes.
3. In the interim, combine the curds, salsa, and one measure of the cheddar. Put aside.

4. Take off the meal dish from the stove and cautiously channel the cooling fluid from the meat. Separate the meat into little pieces. A potato masher works incredible for this. Spread the curds and salsa blend over the heart. Sprinkle the rest of the cheddar to finish everything.
5. Return the meal to the stove and heat for an extra 15-20 minutes until the meat is cooked thoroughly and the cheddar is hot and bubbly.

Nutritional Info (Per Serving): Calories 281; Fat 9 g; Protein 18 g; Carbs 12 g; Fiber 1.2 g

ASPARAGUS AND SALMON DISH

Cook Time: 15 mins | Servings: 3

Ingredients:

- 2 salmon fillets, 6 oz each, skin on
- Sunflower seeds to taste
- 1 lb asparagus, trimmed
- 2 cloves garlic, minced
- 3 tbsps almond butter
- ¼ cup cashew cheese

Directions:
1. Pre-heat your oven to 400°F
2. Line a baking sheet with oil
3. Take a kitchen towel and pat your salmon dry, season as needed
4. Put salmon around baking sheet and arrange asparagus around it
5. Place a pan over medium heat and melt almond butter
6. Add garlic and cook for 3 mins until garlic browns slightly
7. Drizzle sauce over salmon
8. Sprinkle salmon with cheese and bake for 12 mins until salmon looks cooked all the way and is flaky

Nutritional Info (Per Serving): Calories 131; Fat 8 g; Protein 12 g; Carbs 7 g; Fiber 0.8 g

LEMON COD

Cook Time: 18 mins | Servings: 2

Ingredients:

- 4 tbsps almond butter, divided
- 4 thyme sprigs, fresh and divided

- 4 tsps lemon juice, fresh and divided
- 4 cod fillets, 6 oz each
- Sunflower seeds to taste

Directions:

1. Pre-heat your oven to 400 degrees F.
2. Season cod fillets with sunflower seeds on both side.
3. Take four pieces of foil, each foil should be 3 times bigger than fillets.
4. Divide fillets between the foils and top with almond butter, lemon juice, thyme.
5. Fold to form a pouch and transfer pouches to the baking sheet.
6. Bake for 20 mins. Serve.

Nutritional Info (Per Serving): Calories 122; Fat 8 g; Protein 7 g; Carbs 4 g; Fiber 1g

---

CHICKEN COUS COUS

Cook Time: 25 mins | Servings: 4

Ingredients:

- 1-1/2 tsps black pepper, ground
- 1 tsp hot pepper, crushed, dried
- 2 tsps oregano, crushed
- 6 cloves garlic, finely chopped
- 1 cup onion, pureed or finely chopped
- 1/4 cup vinegar
- 3 tbsps brown sugar
- 8 pieces chicken, skinless (4 breasts, 4 drumsticks)

Directions:

1. Preheat oven to 350°F. Wash chicken and pat dry. Combine all Ingredients: except chicken in large bowl. Rub seasonings over chicken and marinate in refrigerator for 6 hours or longer.
2. Space chicken evenly on nonstick or lightly greased baking pan.
3. Cover with aluminum foil and bake for 40 mins. Remove foil and continue baking for an additional 30–40 mins or until the meat can easily be pulled away from the bone with a fork.

Nutritional Info (Per Serving): Calories 113; Fat 4 g; Protein 17 g; Carbs 6 g; Fiber 2g

TURKEY CUTLETS WITH HERBS

Cook Time: 8 mins | Servings: 4

Ingredients:

- 2 tbsp olive oil
- 2 sliced lemons
- 1 package (approx, 1 lb) turkey-breast cutlets
- ½ tsp garlic powder
- 4 cups baby spinach
- ½ cup water
- 2 tsps dried thyme

Directions:

1. In a large skillet over medium-high heat, heat the oil
2. Add about 6 lemon slices to the skillet
3. Sprinkle the turkey-breast cutlets with garlic powder and black pepper
4. Place the turkey cutlets into the skillet and cook for about 3 mins on each side until the turkey is no longer pink and is slightly browned at the edges
5. Remove from heat and divide turkey between 4 plates
6. Add the spinach to the pan along with ½ cup of water and steam, stirring frequently for about 2 mins. Remove the greens and lemons with tongs or a slotted spoon and divide between plates
7. Serve topped with dried thyme

Nutritional Info (Per Serving): Calories 204; Fat 8 g; Protein 30 g; Carbs 8 g; Fiber 4g

Chapter 15. SNACKS AND APPETIZERS RECIPES

CHEDDAR JALAPENO MEATBALLS

Cook Time: 45 mins | **Servings:** 8

Ingredients:

- 1 ½ lb. Ground beef
- 1 large jalapeno, sliced
- 6 oz sharp cheddar, grated
- ½ cup pork rind crumbs
- 1 egg
- 1 tsp chili powder
- 2 tbsp cilantro, chopped
- 1 tsp garlic powder
- ½ tsp cumin
- 1 tsp salt and pepper

Directions:

1. Preheat the oven to 375°F and line a rimmed baking sheet with parchment paper.
2. Mix all ingredients in a blender. Blend on high until well combined. Roll the dough into 1½-inch balls and add to the baking sheet 1 inch apart.
3. Bake for 20 mins. Serve.

Nutritional Info (Per Serving): Calories 368; Fat 24 g; Saturated fat 9.7 g; Protein 33.4 g; Carbs 0.8 g; Fiber 0.3 g; Sugar 1 g.

BACON AND GUACAMOLE FAT BOMBS

Cook Time: 45 mins | **Servings: 6**

Ingredients:

- ¼ cup butter (softened)
- ½ avocado
- 2 garlic cloves, crushed
- ½ small white onion, diced
- 1 small chili pepper, finely chopped
- 1 tbsp lime juice
- 2 tbsp cilantro, chopped
- 4 slices bacon

Directions:

1. Preheat the oven to 375°F and line a baking tray with baking paper. Place the bacon strips on the baking tray.
2. Bake for 15 mins. Remove the tray from the oven and let cool. Crumble the bacon.
3. Cut avocado in half, remove the pit and peel it. Add butter, avocado, chili pepper, cilantro, crushed garlic, and lime juice to a bowl. Season with salt and pepper; mash with a fork until combined.
4. Add onion and mix. Add bacon grease from the baking tray and mix well. Cover with foil and refrigerate for 30 mins.
5. Shape the guacamole mixture into 6 balls. Roll each ball into the bacon pieces and place on a tray. Serve.

Nutritional Info (Per Serving): Calories 156; Fat 15.2 g; Saturated fat 6.8 g; Protein 3.4 g; Carbs 1.4 g; Fiber 1.3 g; Sugar 0.5 g.

BUFFALO CHICKEN SAUSAGE BALLS

Cook Time: 40 mins | Servings: 12 balls

Ingredients:

- 3 tbsps coconut flour
- 24 oz. bulk chicken sausage
- 1 cup cheddar cheese, shredded
- 1 cup almond flour
- ½ cup Buffalo wing sauce
- ½ tsp cayenne
- 1 tsp salt
- ½ tsp pepper
- 2 garlic cloves, minced
- 1 tsp dried dill
- ⅓ cup mayonnaise
- ⅓ cup almond milk, unsweetened
- ½ tsp dried parsley
- ¼ cup bleu cheese, crumbled
- ½ tsp salt
- ½ tsp pepper

Directions:

1. Preheat the oven to 350°F and line 2 baking sheets with parchment paper.
2. Mix cheddar cheese, sausage, almond flour, coconut flour, buffalo sauce, cayenne, salt, and pepper in a bowl and mix well until combined.

3. Roll the mixture into 1-inch balls and place on the baking sheets 1 inch apart—Bake for 25 mins.
4. Mix mayo, almond milk, garlic, parsley, dill, salt, and pepper in a bowl. Mix well and add bleu cheese in. Mix well.
5. Serve balls with the sauce.

Nutritional Info (Per Serving): Calories 255; Fat 19.3 g; Saturated fat 4.7 g; Protein 15.3 g; Carbs 2.5 g; Fiber 1.7 g; Sugar 5 g.

COCONUT CHOCOLATE CHIP COOKIES

Cook Time: 30 mins | Servings: 6

Ingredients:

- 1 egg
- 3/4 cup coconut shredded
- 1 ¼ cup almond flour
- 1 tsp baking powder
- 1/2 cup swerve sweetener
- 1/2 cup vanilla extract
- 1/2 cup chocolate chips, sugar-free
- 1/2 cup butter
- ¼ tsp fine salt

Directions:

1. Preheat the oven to 325°F and line a baking sheet with parchment paper.
2. Mix coconut, almond flour, baking powder, and salt in a bowl.
3. Mix butter with sweetener in a separate bowl. Beat in egg and vanilla. Stir to combine. Add this mixture to the flour mixture and beat it well. Add in the chocolate chips.
4. Shape the dough into 1½-inch balls. Place on the baking sheet 2 inches apart. Press each ball to ¼-inch thick.
5. Bake for 15 mins. Remove from the oven and cool completely. Serve.

Nutritional Info (Per Serving): Calories 268; Fat 17.4 g; Saturated fat 10.3 g; Protein 12 g; Carbs 12 g; Fiber 1 g; Sugar 10 g.

OAT-FREE PORRIDGE

Cook Time: 5 mins | Servings: 1

Ingredients:

- 2 tbsp unsweetened coconut, shredded
- ½ cup of water
- 2 tbsp hemp hearts

- 2 tbsp almond flour
- 1 tbsp chia seeds
- 1 tbsp golden flaxseed meal
- ¼ tsp granulated stevia
- ½ tsp pure vanilla extract
- 1 pinch salt

Directions:

1. Add all ingredients except vanilla to a saucepan.
2. Cook over low heat for 5 mins, stirring constantly. Add in the vanilla. Serve.

Nutritional Info (Per Serving): Calories 453; Fat 36 g; Protein 18 g; Carbs 5 g; Fiber 10 g; Sugar 1 g.

KETO BOWL

Cook Time: 30 mins | Servings: 1

Ingredients:

- 1 egg
- ¼ cup cheddar cheese, shredded
- 2 cups radishes
- 3½ oz. ground sausage
- ¼ tsp pink Himalayan salt
- ¼ tsp black pepper

Directions:

1. Cook sausage in a pan over medium-high heat until done. Remove sausage from the pan and set aside.
2. Cut radishes into small pieces and add to the pan. Season well. Cook radishes for 12 mins.
3. Fry the egg the way you want and set it aside. Layer the radishes with sausage on a plate, top with egg and cheese. Serve.

Nutritional Info (Per Serving): Calories 617; Fat 49 g; Saturated fat 11.1 g; Protein 32 g; Carbs 4 g; Fiber 3 g; Sugar 5 g.

SAUSAGE AND PEPPERS

Cook Time: 50 mins | Servings: 4

Ingredients:

- 1½ tsp olive oil
- 1 green bell pepper, chopped
- 1 red bell pepper, chopped
- ½ cup mozzarella cheese, grated
- 10 oz. sausage
- Salt, black pepper, to taste

Directions:

1. Preheat the oven to 450°F and grease a medium-sized dish with cooking spray.
2. Add peppers to the baking dish and toss with 1 tsp olive oil and add salt and black pepper on top—Bake for 20 mins.
3. Heat remaining olive oil on a pan and add the sausages. Cook over medium-high heat for 12 mins.
4. Cut sausages into pieces. Add the sausages to the baking pan with the peppers—Bake for 5 more mins.
5. Remove the dish from the oven, turn the oven to broil. Add the mozzarella over the peppers and sausages. Broil for 2 mins. Serve.

Nutritional Info (Per Serving): Calories 246; Fat 13 g; Saturated fat 5 g; Protein 26 g; Carbs 4 g; Fiber 1 g; Sugar 2 g.

CHOCOLATE MINT SMOOTHIE

Cook Time: 5 mins | Servings: 1

Ingredients:

- 2 scoops of chocolate collagen protein
- 2 tbsps coconut, shredded
- ½ cup of coconut milk
- 1 tbsp cacao butter, crushed
- 1 cup of water
- 4 mint leaves
- ½ cup ice
- ½ a frozen avocado

Directions:

1. Add all the ingredients *except* for shredded coconut and collagen protein to a blender.
2. Blend on high for about 45 seconds. Then add collagen protein to a blender and blend for 5 seconds more.
3. Top chocolate mint avocado smoothie with coconut flakes. Enjoy!

Nutritional Info (Per Serving): Calories 552; Fat 44 g; Saturated fat 25 g; Protein 26 g; Carbs 1 g; Fiber 9 g; Sugar 2 g.

BACON AND EGG MUFFINS

Cooking time: 25 mins | Servings: 12

Ingredients:

- 8 eggs
- 8 bacon slices
- ⅔ cup green onion, chopped
- Cooking spray
- 8 muffins

Directions:

1. Coat the muffin tin with nonstick cooking spray and preheat the oven to 350°F.
2. Add bacon to a large pan and cook over medium heat until crisp. Transfer to a plate lined with paper towels. Let cool and then chop into small pieces.
3. Add eggs to a bowl and whisk well. Then add green onions and cooked bacon. Mix until everything is well-combined.
4. Add the mixture to the muffin tin. Bake for about 20-25 mins, until edges are golden brown.
5. Let the muffins cool and enjoy bacon and egg breakfast muffins.

Nutritional Info (Per Serving): Calories 158; Fat 13.3 g; Saturated fat 1.7 g; Protein 8 g; Carbs 1 g; Fiber 0 g; Sugar 1 g.

LOW CARB WAFFLES

Cooking Time: 15 mins | Servings: 1

Ingredients:

- 3 egg whites
- 2 tablespoons unsweetened almond milk
- 2 tablespoons coconut flour
- ½ teaspoon baking powder
- Sweetener, optional

Directions:

1. Whip 2 of the egg whites using a hand mixer or egg beater.
2. Stir in the coconut flour, milk, baking powder, sweetener, and 1 egg white.
3. Heat up the waffle iron and grease with a nonstick spray.
4. Pour in the batter and cook in the waffle iron for 3 to 4 minutes until browned.
5. Pull it out and serve.

Nutritional Info (Per Serving): Calories: 264 Fat: 22g Protein: 14g Carbs: 6g

VANILLA AND MARSHMALLOW SMOOTHIE

Cooking Time: 25 mins |Servings: 2

Ingredients:

- ½ cup of coconut milk
- 1 cup of water
- 3 cups of ice
- 2 tbsp. of chia
- 1 tsp. vanilla extract
- 2 tbsp. collage hydrosol
- honey to taste

Directions:

1. Place the ingredients in your blender or food processor.
2. Blend until creamy smooth. Serve.

Nutritional Info (Per Serving): Calories 258; Fat 18.3 g; Saturated fat 1.9 g; Protein 8 g; Carbs 18 g; Fiber 0 g; Sugar 4 g.

PUMPKIN ALMOND PANCAKES

Cooking Time: 10 mins |Servings: 2

Ingredients:

- 4 oz. vanilla whey protein powder
- ½ cup pumpkin puree, canned
- Four eggs, beaten
- 1 tsp. Double-acting baking powder, sodium aluminum sulfate
- 1 cup creamed cottage cheese
- ¼ cup almond flour, blanched
- ½ teaspoon pumpkin pie spice

- ¼ cup whole grain soy flour, dry

Directions:

1. Combine the protein powder, pumpkin pie spice, almond flour, baking powder, and soy flour in a bowl.
2. Add the remaining ingredients and mix until well blended.
3. Grease a skillet using butter.
4. Pour ¼ cup of the batter into the skillet and cook over medium heat. Once bubbles form in the middle, flip the pancakes over and cook until firm.
5. Repeat the procedure with the remaining batter.

Nutritional Info (Per Serving): Calories 183; Fat 8.5 g; Protein 21 g; Carbs 4.8 g; Fiber 2 g; Sugar 5 g.

EGGS WITH SALSA AND AVOCADO

Cooking Time: 12 mins | Servings: 1

Ingredients:

- Two eggs
- ½ Avocado, peeled, deseeded, and sliced.
- 1 oz. salsa
- 4 oz. turkey sausage
- 1/8 cantaloupe melon, sliced

Directions:

1. Fry eggs in a pan.
2. Arrange Avocado on the bottom of a plate. Place eggs on top, followed by salsa.
3. Cook sausage over high heat until browned on all sides. Serve with egg stack and cantaloupe slices.

Nutritional Info (Per Serving): Calories 474; Fat 8.5 g; Protein 36 g; Carbs 14.8 g; Fiber 5.2 g; Sugar 3.5 g.

BAKED EGGPLANT PUREE

Cooking Time: 40 mins | Servings: 1

Ingredients:

- 16 tomatoes
- One cucumber

- 2 Tsp. ground pepper
- 2 large eggplants
- One clove (s) garlic.
- Ground coriander

Directions:

1. Preheat the oven to high temperature. Make deep cuts in the eggplants and place them on a baking tray. Bake until smooth, about 30 to 40 minutes.
2. Let them cool until they can be manipulated, about 15 minutes for large aubergines and picas (or briefly pass through the blender or food processor), and place in a medium bowl.
3. Mix with oil, garlic, and cilantro. Salt and pepper to taste. Serve the mixture to accompany raw vegetable snacks such as cucumber sticks or cherry tomatoes.

Nutritional Info (Per Serving): Calories 155; Fat 11.5 g; Protein 8 g; Carbs 1.8 g; Fiber 2 g; Sugar 5 g.

AVOCADO SALSA

Cooking Time: 2 mins | Servings: 1

Ingredients:

- 1 Red tomato
- ⅛ cup fresh cilantro, rough chopped
- 1 Red onion, diced
- ½ jalapeno pepper, diced
- 2 Avocadoes, diced
- 2-3 Tbsp. fresh lime juice
- Pinch of salt and new ground black pepper

Directions:

1. Chop all the vegetables.
2. Add them to a bowl.
3. Squeeze in the lime juice. Season with salt and pepper. Stir.
4. Refrigerate for 30 minutes. Serve.

Nutritional Info (Per Serving): Calories 75; Fat 5.5 g; Protein 1.6 g; Carbs 4.8 g; Fiber 3.2 g; Sugar 4.5 g.

Chapter 16. VEGETARIAN RECIPES

ZUCCHINI NOODLE SALAD

Cook Time: 15 mins | Servings: 8 cups

Ingredients:

- 8 oz. mozzarella pearls
- 1 oz. basil, chopped
- 4 zucchinis, spiralized
- 4 oz. cherry tomatoes, sliced in half
- 3 tbsp red wine vinegar
- ¼ cup extra virgin olive oil
- 1 tbsp lemon juice
- ¼ tsp garlic powder
- ½ tsp salt
- ¼ tsp pepper

Directions:

1. Whisk red wine, oil, lemon juice, garlic powder, salt, and pepper in a bowl.
2. Add the remaining ingredients to a bowl and add dressing on top. Toss well to combine. Serve.

Nutritional Info (Per Serving): Calories 186; Fat 13 g; Saturated fat 4 g; Protein 7 g; Carbs 3 g; Fiber 1 g; Sugar 3 g.

CAULIFLOWER RISOTTO

Cook Time: 10 mins | Servings: 2

Ingredients:

- 1 tbsp. olive oil
- 2 garlic cloves, minced
- 4 baby Bella mushrooms, diced
- 1 cup chicken broth
- 2 cups riced cauliflower
- ¼ cup parmesan cheese
- ¼ cup heavy cream
- 1 tsp. tarragon

- Pinch of salt and pepper

Directions:

1. In a blender, process the cauliflower until rice-like consistency.
2. In a skillet, heat the olive oil. Sauté the garlic mushrooms for 3 minutes.
3. Pour in the chicken broth and cauliflower. Stir well. Simmer 5 minutes.
4. Once the liquid has cooked away, add the parmesan cheese and tarragon, salt, and pepper. Stir well. Stir in the cream. Keep stirring until the cheese has melted.
5. Serve hot.

Nutritional Info (Per Serving): Calories 246; Fat 21 g; Protein 6.5 g; Carbs 8.9 g

MACARONI AND CHEESE

Cook Time: 30 mins | Servings: 8

Ingredients:

- 2 cups macaroni
- 2 cups onions, chopped
- 2 cups evaporated fat-free milk
- 1 medium egg, beaten
- 1/4 tsp black pepper
- 1-1/4 cups low-fat cheddar cheese, finely shredded
- nonstick cooking spray, as needed

Directions:

1. Preheat oven to 350° F.
2. Lightly spray saucepan with nonstick cooking spray. Add onions to saucepan and sauté for about 3 mins.
3. In another bowl, combine macaroni, onions, and the rest of the ingredients and mix thoroughly.
4. Transfer mixture into casserole dish.
5. Bake for 20 mins or until bubbly. Let stand for 10 mins before serving.

Nutritional Info (Per Serving): Calories 200; Fat 4 g; Protein 12 g; Carbs 29 g

PESTO AND GOAT CHEESE TERRINE

Cook Time: 25 mins | Servings: 10

Ingredients:

- 1/4 cup toasted and chopped pine nuts
- ½ cup heavy cream

- 10 oz crumbled goat cheese
- 5 chopped sundried tomatoes
- 3 tbsp basil pesto
- 1 tbsp toasted and chopped pine nuts

Directions:

1. Mix the goat cheese with the heavy cream and stir using your mixer
2. Spoon half of this mix into a lined bowl and spread
3. Put the pesto on top and spread
4. Put another layer of cheese and then add sundried tomatoes and 1/4 cup pine nuts
5. Spread the final layer of cheese and top with 1 tbsp pine nuts
6. Refrigerate for about 20 mins
7. Flip upside down on a plate and serve cold.

Nutritional Info (Per Serving): Calories 240; Fat 12 g; Protein 12 g; Carbs 5 g

LENTILS WITH BROWN RICE

Cook Time: 30 mins | Servings: 4

Ingredients:

For lentils and kale

- 1 cup brown lentils, rinsed
- 1/8 tsp ground black pepper

For brown rice

- 1 cup instant brown rice, uncooked (for quinoa, follow cooking instructions on box)
- 1/2 tsp dried basil
- For onion
- 2 tbsps olive oil
- 2 cups onion, diced
- 1/8 tsp ground black pepper

Directions:

1. Rinse lentils thoroughly in a fine wire colander and remove any stones or debris.
2. In a 4-quart saucepan, cover lentils with 2-1/2 cups of water. Add salt and pepper. Cover, and bring to a boil over high heat. Reduce heat. Simmer for 20 mins
3. In another saucepan, bring 2 cups of water to a boil. Add rice, salt, and basil. Cover, and cook for 10 mins. Set aside.
4. In a medium sauté pan, warm olive oil over medium heat and add onion, salt, and pepper. Cook and stir until the onion pieces become soft and dark brown (caramelized), but not burnt. If the onions start to stick to the pan, add a few drops of water and scrape the onions

loose. Keep cooking until onions are completely caramelized (about 10–15 mins total). Remove from pan and set aside.

5. When the lentils are tender, but not mushy, mix the lentils, and caramelized onions in the sauté pan and stir.

6. To serve, put 1 cup of the lentil mixture, in the form of a ring, on each of four dinner plates. Fill the center of each ring with one-fourth of the brown rice. Serve immediately.

7. Roasted and chopped pine nuts

8. Mix the goat cheese with the heavy cream and stir using your mixer

Nutritional Info (Per Serving): Calories 456; Fat 9 g; Protein 21 g; Carbs 77 g

BRUSSELS SPROUTS CHIPS

Cook Time: 15-20 mins | Servings: 4

Ingredients:

- 1 lb. Brussels sprouts washed and dried, ends trimmed
- 1 tsp salt
- 2 tbsps extra virgin olive oil
- Smoked paprika, for serving

Directions:

1. Preheat the oven to 400°F
2. Peel the outer leaves of the Brussels sprouts and discard them. Add the sprouts to a bowl.
3. Drizzle with oil and toss well to coat in oil. Season with salt. Spread on a baking sheet evenly in one layer.
4. Bake for about 12-15 mins. Take them out from the oven and let them cool.
5. Sprinkle with more salt if you want. Serve topped with smoked paprika.

Nutritional Info (Per Serving): Calories 104; Fat 7 g; Saturated fat 1.4 g; Protein 3 g; Carbs 5 g; Fiber 4 g; Sugar 1 g.

CHEESY CRACKERS

Cook Time: 45 mins | Servings: 8

Ingredients:

- ½ cup flax meal
- 1 cup almond flour
- 2 tbsp whole psyllium husks

- 1 cup of water
- 1 cup Parmesan cheese, grated
- 1 tsp salt
- ¼ tsp black pepper

Directions:

1. Mix flax meal, almond flour, psyllium, salt, and pepper in a bowl. Add the cheese to it and mix well. Add water and mix well. Let rest for 15 mins.
2. Preheat the oven to 320°F and divide the dough into 2 parts.
3. Place half of the dough on parchment paper. Place another piece of parchment paper on top and roll the dough out until thin.
4. Cut the dough into 16 equal pieces. Repeat the process with the remaining dough.
5. Bake for 45 mins. Serve.

Nutritional info (per serving): Calories 169; Fat 13.4 g; Saturated fat 2.7 g; Protein 8.4 g; Carbs 1.7 g; Fiber 4.5 g; Sugar 0.8 g.

ALMOND BARK

Cooking time: 15 mins | Servings: 20

Ingredients:

- 4 oz. cocoa butter
- ½ cup Swerve sweetener
- ½ tsp vanilla extract
- 2 tbsps water
- ¾ cup cocoa powder
- 1 tbsp butter
- ½ cup powdered Swerve sweetener
- 1½ cups roasted almonds, unsalted
- 2½ oz. unsweetened chocolate, chopped
- ¼ tsp sea salt

Directions:

1. Add 2 tbsp water and ½ cup Swerve sweetener to a saucepan. Bring the mixture to a light boil, stirring occasionally. Cook for about 8 to 9 mins until the mixture darkens.
2. Turn the heat off and whisk in 1 tbsp butter. Add 1½ cups roasted almonds and toss well until coated. Then stir in 2 pinches of salt.
3. Spread almonds onto a parchment-lined baking sheet. Add 4 oz. cocoa butter and 2½ oz. unsweetened chocolate to a large saucepan. Melt over medium heat and stir until smooth.
4. Stir in ¾ cup cocoa powder and ½ cup powdered Swerve sweetener until smooth. Turn the heat off and stir in ½ tsp vanilla extract.

5. Reserve 4 tbsp of almonds and keep them aside. Add leftover almonds to the chocolate mixture and stir well.
6. Spread chocolate-almond mixture out onto the same baking sheet. Top with reserved ¼ cups of almonds and sprinkle with salt.
7. Chill for about 3 hours and then break into chunks. Serve right away!

Nutritional Info (Per Serving): Calories 144; Fat 14 g; Saturated fat 1.3 g; Protein 13 g; Carbs 2 g; Fiber 3 g; Sugar 10 g.

DEVILED EGGS

Cook Time: 20 mins | Servings: 6

Ingredients:

- 12 eggs
- 8 oz full-fat cream cheese
- 1/2 cup butter
- ¼ tsp fine salt and pepper

Directions:

1. Add eggs to cold water, bring to a boil and cook for 10 mins. Drain and add to cold water; let rest for 1-2 mins. Peel the eggs.
2. Cut eggs in half lengthwise and scoop out the yolks. Add yolks to the bowl.
3. Slice cream cheese and add to the bowl with yolks. Blend well. Add in the salt and pepper and beat well.
4. Fill egg whites with the yolk mixture. Add seasoning son top. Serve.

Nutritional Info (Per Serving): Calories 277; Fat 22.6 g; Protein 14.9 g; Carbs 3.1 g; Fiber 0.2 g; Sugar 1.6 g.

CHEESE PANCAKES

Cook Time: 15 mins | Servings: 2

Ingredients:

- 2 eggs
- 4 oz. cream cheese
- ½ tsp baking powder
- ¼ cup almond flour
- ¼ tsp fine salt

- Cooking spray

Directions:

1. Mix eggs, flour, cream cheese, baking powder, and salt in a blender and blend until smooth.
2. Heat a frying pan over medium heat and grease with cooking spray. Add 3 tbsp of the batter. Cook for 3 mins. Flip and cook for 2 more mins. Transfer to a plate.
3. Repeat with the remaining batter. Serve.

Nutritional Info (Per Serving): Calories 329; Fat 30.2 g; Protein 10.1 g; Carbs 4.2 g; Fiber 1.3 g; Sugar 2.9 g.

Chapter 17. 28 Day Meal Plan

DAYS	LUNCH	SNACK	DINNER
1	Swiss Chard Omelet	Yogurt with Fruits and oats	Black-Bean and Vegetable Burrito
2	Shrimp Pasta Primavera	Italian Cheese Sticks	Baked Eggs In Avocado
3	Garlic Parmesan Wings	Chickpeas Hummus	Black-Bean Soup and croutons
4	Southwestern Chicken and Pasta	Quinoa and Date Bowl	Loaded Baked Sweet Potatoes
5	Basil and Tomato Baked Eggs	Zingy Onion and Thyme Crackers	Chicken and Broccoli Stir-Fry
6	Cool Mushroom Munchies and rice	Ham Toast	Chicken Fajitas
7	Italian Meatballs and whole pasta	Crunchy Flax and Almond Crackers	Honey-Mustard Chicken
8	Ground Beef And Green Beans	Hearty Pineapple Oatmeal	Grilled Chicken, Avocado, and Apple Salad
9	Moroccan Lamb Tajine	Banana and nuts Porridge	Turkey Cutlets with Herbs
10	Curry Lamb Shanks	Delightful Berry Quinoa Bowl	Roast Salmon with Roasted Asparagus
11	Worthwhile Balsamic Beef	Tomatoes Ground Beef And Green Beans And	Crispy Chicken Egg Rolls
12	Garlic Parmesan Wings and rice	Smoothie	Cilantro-Lime Tilapia Tacos
13	Poke Bowls Rice and Shrimps	Cinnamon and Pumpkin Porridge	Lemon-Parsley Baked Flounder and Brussels Sprouts

14	Lamb Spare Ribs	Fresh Fruits and nuts	Pan-Seared Scallops
15	Crispy Chicken Egg Rolls	Tomatoes and Garlic Toast	Baked Cod Packets with Broccoli
16	Mushroom Bacon Skillet	Healthy Granola Bowl	Garlic Salmon and Snap Peas In Foil
17	Low-Carb Zucchini Lasagna Rolls	Brussels Sprouts Chips	Southwestern Chicken and Pasta
18	Buffalo Chicken Salad Wrap	Guacamole	Italian Salad
19	Low-Carb Chili	Almond Bark	Chicken Sliders
20	Broccoli Sticks	Cheese Pancakes	Black-Eyed Peas and Greens Power Salad
21	Ceasar Salad	Smoothie Bowl	Butternut-Squash Macaroni
22	Marinated beef Kebabs	Bacon Muffin	Pasta with Tomatoes and Peas
23	Salmon and Cauliflower rice	Chocolate Mint Smoothie	Steak tacos
24	Pesto And Goat Cheese Terrine	Green Crackers	Portobello-Mushroom Cheeseburgers
25	Vanilla Sweet Potato Porridge	Cheesy Crackers	Pork Salad with Walnuts and Peaches
26	Sausage and peppers	Special Cucumber Cups	Baked Chickpea-and-Rosemary Omelet
27	Healthy Vegetable Fried Rice	Ham Tost	Deviled Eggs
28	Greek beef	Yogurt and fruits	Asian pork tenderloin

CONCLUSION

Intermittent fasting is a broad term for an eating pattern in which food consumption is limited to less than eight hours per day. Fasting periods are typically 16 or 24 hours in length. It is not about "starving" oneself but rather about sticking to an eight-hour eating schedule.

Intermittent fasting has numerous advantages, including weight loss and improved insulin sensitivity. Intermittent fasting has also been shown in studies to help reduce inflammation and fight chronic disease. Intermittent fasting, regardless of age or current health status, can be beneficial for some people. These advantages are as follows:

1. Weight Loss Has Increased

Studies have shown intermittent rapidity to help people lose weight rapidly. At the same time, no one knows why; some theories include a lack of appetite, hormonal changes, and a feeling of fullness from fasting.

2. Insulin Sensitivity Has Improved

Intermittent fasting studies have shown that the body's sensitivity to insulin can be increased, blood glucose levels potentially reduced, and insulin resistance improved.

3. Reduced Chronic Disease Risk

Several studies have found that eating patterns such as intermittent fasting can help prevent chronic diseases such as type 2 diabetes and heart disease by aiding in weight management, lowering oxidative stress, decreasing inflammation, improving physical performance, and much more.

4. Lipid Profile Enhancement

Intermittent fasting was shown in studies to improve the lipid profile with an increase in HDL and LDL cholesterol, which shows it reduces the risk of cardiovascular disease.

5. C-Reactive Protein levels are lower.

A blood protein marker of inflammation-causing or aggravating diseases such as type 2 diabetes, heart disease, and certain cancers is the CRP. C-reactive protein (CRP). Intermittent quicking decreases CRP levels in the blood.

6. Physical Performance Enhancement

Intermittent rapidity has been demonstrated in studies to increase physical performance and perhaps increase lean muscle mass and decrease fat. It makes sense because regular exercise increases the production of new muscle cells, while fasting reduces the demand for food and makes it more energy-producing.

7. Better Mental Health

According to research, intermittent fasting may improve cognition and mental health. In some cases, intermittent fasting has been linked to improved mood, less depression, and fewer anxiety symptoms. It's also worth noting that many people who fast regularly claim to feel better overall than when they don't eat at all!

8. Cancer Risk is Reduced

According to research, eating patterns such as intermittent fasting can reduce the risk of certain types of cancer, such as breast cancer.

9. Reduced Risk of Dementia and Alzheimer's Disease

Most studies on intermittent fasting have focused on people aged 60 and up, but it's worth noting that intermittent fasting may also help prevent diseases like dementia and Alzheimer's. Some studies have discovered a link between long-term intermittent fasting (eating fewer than five meals per day and fasting for more than 20 hours between meals) and a lower risk of cognitive decline and Alzheimer's disease.

10. Life expectancy

Several studies have found that eating patterns such as intermittent fasting may increase lifespan, though it is unclear how this occurs.

What Is the Process of Intermittent Fasting?

Intermittent is a broad term that refers to a variety of eating patterns and time frames. The two most common plans are intermittent daily fasting (alternating 24-hour periods of eating with 24-hour periods of not eating) and the 5:2 diet. Women consume less than 500 calories per day for two days per week (usually Monday and Thursday).

In general, Intermittent Fasting consists of two phases: fasting and feeding. When we fast, our bodies must rely on stored energy to keep us alive; this is referred to as the ketogenic stage. The less fuel there is, the more severe the ketosis and the less we can eat. The goal of using an intermittent fasting schedule is to reach a state of ketosis in which fat burning takes precedence over carbohydrate burning as the primary driver of energy production. However, some people prefer to consume 50-60% carbs for breakfast to not run out of energy too quickly.

Some people enjoy a snack meal after their fast because they are hungry but have not yet consumed enough calories to be in proper starvation mode. Study of behavioral nutrition and physical activities in the International Journal published in April 2014 found that eating breakfast created more feelings of completeness than breakfast savings and improved cognitive tasks performance.

I hope you enjoyed reading this book at least as much as I enjoyed writing it. But even more, I hope that this reading may have been a push for you to take action because you know, you won't get fitter, healthier, or thinner just by reading a book.

Again, I want to stress my main point about this diet: of course, you now have some technical information, some ideas, some hints about a better lifestyle related to intermittent fasting. And this is great. Though, the main thing about this, or any other diet, is not how it technically works. It is that you should enjoy it. You should visualize your goal and then love the journey; whatever the reasons behind your decision to take this path, they all are the same reason: you love yourself, and you want to act like it.

So that is what you have to do, loving yourself, taking care of yourself: you are not following a diet, you're following yourself.

THANK YOU

FOR PURCHASING MY BOOK.
I HOPE YOU ENJOYED IT!
IF SO REMEMBER TO LEAVE A REVIEW,
I WILL APPRECIATE IT VERY MUCH ❤

Made in the USA
Las Vegas, NV
15 October 2021